The Book of
GAMES AND WARM UPS
FOR GROUP LEADERS

2nd Edition

LEO RUTHERFORD

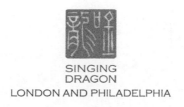

SINGING
DRAGON
LONDON AND PHILADELPHIA

This edition published in 2015
by Singing Dragon
an imprint of Jessica Kingsley Publishers
73 Collier Street
London N1 9BE, UK
and
400 Market Street, Suite 400
Philadelphia, PA 19106, USA

www.singingdragon.com

First edition published by Gale Centre Publications in 1994

Front cover image source: Shutterstock®

Library of Congress Cataloging in Publication Data
A CIP catalog record for this book is available from the Library of Congress

British Library Cataloguing in Publication Data
A CIP catalogue record for this book is available from the British Library

ISBN 978 1 84819 235 5
eISBN 978 0 85701 184 8

Printed and bound in Great Britain

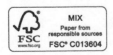

Contents

Acknowledgements

Many people contributed to what became Play-World! First, the teachers I was lucky enough to come across: Gabrielle Roth, who got me into dancing, out of my head and back into my body at the tender age of 42; Keith Johnstone, both through his wonderful book *Impro* and at a workshop I attended, who inspired me about the value of theatre improvisation; Chungliang Al Huang, who helped me find the Tai-chi spirit of effortless play; Joan Halifax, Harley Swiftdeer and Prem Das, who taught me about the Medicine Way of seeing and being in the world; Will Schutz, Director of the Holistic Studies programme at Antioch University, San Francisco, who pushed my buttons, especially the ones I didn't want to own; Marilyn Kreigel, who helped and guided me through my degree course; the Antioch Holy House crew of San Francisco, who supported and helped me through difficult times of growth and change; Linda Riebel, who has been a friend for all seasons; and so many other wonderful people I met along the way. I also want to acknowledge the work of the New Games Foundation and Matt Wienstein of Playfair, who are pioneers in the field of non-competitive play. Then the Play-World gang of 1983–1987: Trisha Wood, Ian Kalman, Bill Downey and Pete Miller, who co-led and helped in numerous ways; Dave Sumeray and Joe Cymrank, who kept the outrageous creativity content high; and all the other people who participated in multifarious Play-World events and helped to make so many great times. Jane Burke, who put my original scruffy manuscript onto disk, Bill Downey for enormous help with the manuscript, Bruce Anderson, Trisha Wood, Lesley Bennington, Tony Whieldon, Jane Henriques, Hilary Wainer, Bianca Benjamin, Susan Lever and David Sumeray, who all ploughed through it and gave me helpful comments and suggestions, and Elsien and Derek Gale who had enough faith to publish this book.

Second edition: Thanks to Jessica Kingsley and the team at Singing Dragon.

Preface

Every one of us has been a child, and when we were children we could do many things we can't do now. We could lose ourselves in play quite easily and many of us had imaginary friends who were very real to us and kept us company. To us, the world was a magical, multi-dimensional place of extraordinary joy and beauty and sometimes of excruciating sadness and grief. It was a world full of many forms of life, from people to animals to flowers to teddy bears. But as we grew up we were taught to see only the consensus reality of the adult world and to 'leave behind childish things'. Sadly, most of us left behind childlike things as well, including much of our ability to enter the 'Magic Kingdom of Play'.

This book is about ways of retrieving lost pieces of ourselves so that we can become whole again. In the process of growing up and of becoming 'civilised', most of us lose a lot of our natural childlike ability to play. Of course many people play football, cricket, tennis, Monopoly, Trivial Pursuit, bingo and a multitude of other such games, but all these games are competitive. They are mostly about winning, about achieving and proving oneself – as if proof is needed that one is a person of worth! This is not 'play' in the sense I mean. It is not the natural, spontaneous, unpremeditated, non-manipulative play of childhood that happens in the moment of *now*. When we lose the ability to be in the process of life, we tend to become obsessed with the end result of winning or losing – fear of success can also be an obsession.

We have been educated to live in the world through our left brain – our logical, rational, counting brain – while our right brain – the intuitive, holistic, visionary side of us – is reduced in importance and all too often almost forgotten. One great way to reactivate this aspect of ourselves is through non-competitive play, and that includes interactive games, dancing, creating theatre, drawing and singing.

Play, fantasy, imagination, experimentation, adventure, free expression of possibilities and the ability to create according to vision are central qualities of a human being. The original meaning of the word 'human' comes from two words: 'hu', which means divine, and 'man', which means mortal. Thus the ancients who created language tell us we are divine mortals. We are here on planet Earth, the 'School for Souls', to learn, experiment, make mistakes and have adventures; in a word, to play! True play is activity that is spontaneous, without predetermination, unplanned. Play keeps us young at heart, fresh of mind, healthy in body and youthful in spirit. We are playful, imaginative explorers of the external world of things and also the internal world of consciousness. We are aspects of the cosmos looking at itself.

Physicist Brian Swimme says that biologists studying humans and chimpanzees have found that they share over

98 per cent similarity in their gene pools, yet it is obvious that behavioural differences are enormous. He says:

> Current thinking locates the difference between humans and other primates in the ability of the human to make play its dominant activity throughout a lifetime. Unique among species, the human makes exploration, surprising discoveries, experimentations and above all – learning – the central activity of life itself.

(Swimme 1984)

Side by side with play goes laughter. Humour is the great transformer and it is ever-present with adventurous play. It is the means of changing tragedy into comedy, pain into pleasure, confusion into understanding. Humour is a release mechanism for tension and aggression. It is a means by which we can see the other side of something, the forest from the trees, truth out of a maze of confusion. To quote something I heard Professor Arnold Keyserling say: 'A spiritual truth is like a joke you have just understood.' Healthy laughter leads to understanding and growth.

Many kings, queens and emperors of old had their jesters. The jester was able, through humour, to tell the king truths that he would not have been able to hear from any other source without loss of face. The honoured tradition of the jester lives on in comedians who tell society and its rulers' unpleasant truths. They poke out the hypocrisies, lies, pontifications and pomposity through which we can all get conned if we don't watch out!

Laughter and tears are two aspects of one energy. The expression 'I laughed till I cried' expresses a literal truth: the ultimate of a good belly laughing session is tears rolling down cheeks. Likewise at the end of a good cry, when one has truly let go, there is nothing left to do but to laugh. To laugh and to cry is healthy; to dam up the natural flow of either (and many of us, men especially, have been taught not to cry) is to dam up life energy. Laughter and play are the greatest medicine and have been practised by humans ever since we have been on this planet!

In his book, *Anatomy of an Illness* (1981), Norman Cousins tells that in 1964 he was struck down with a rare disease and was in constant pain, barely able to move. He was in a dull and depressing hospital and was given a 1 in 500 chance of survival. He checked himself out of the hospital into a hotel room and arranged the hire of a film projector and his favourite comic films: The Marx Brothers, Laurel and Hardy, Chaplin, and early *Candid Camera* TV shows. He found that ten minutes of belly laughter brought him about two hours of pain-free sleep and that sedimentation readings taken before and after showed a positive change in body chemistry. More recent research has shown that laughter releases endorphins into the blood stream, which are the body's natural pain-killers. Laughter also helped Norman to feel that life was worthwhile and thus mobilise his body's inner healer. He quotes in his book a meeting with Dr Albert Schweitzer in Africa, when he was taken to see a local witch doctor in action. Schweitzer tells him there is:

> a secret that doctors have carried around inside them ever since Hippocrates. Each patient carries his own doctor inside him... We are at our best when we give the doctor who resides within each patient a chance to go to work.

> (Cousins 1981, p.69)

In November 1982, shortly before I returned to England at the end of five years of living in the USA, I attended a conference entitled 'The Healing Power of Laughter and Play' aboard the *Queen Mary*, moored at Long Beach, California. Norman Cousins was the keynote speaker and 18 years after being pronounced terminally ill, he was in fine health and excellent humour!

My own journey has been much guided and influenced by the teachings of the Medicine Wheel from the Native Americans. In their tradition, the Heyeokah, or Contrary, is a person who holds a special place, and whose task is to show truth through humour – to hold up an upside down mirror to the world, and to help people keep their vision, their sense of worth and connection with the Creator even in the darkest and most difficult of times. I have met many native people, including some wonderful grandfathers and grandmothers who were around 100 years old, living in poor circumstances from the point of view of material wealth, but they have all been rich in humour and wisdom, and they most certainly knew how to play.

My thesis is that laughter and play are basic human needs, that they feed the soul, help us transform the pain of living, mobilise our inner resources, guide us to know ourselves better and help us to actualise our potential.

In 1983, after moving to London, I founded Play-World to transform my ideas into action. Play-World is a name I coined for the workshops (play shops) which I started in the October of that year. I wanted to approach the whole therapeutic life change process from the opposite end of most psychotherapy approaches. Instead of bringing people together to find out 'what's wrong', I wanted to bring people together to celebrate and have fun and extend themselves in creative, interactive, imaginative, adventurous activity. Life issues and personal problems will then show themselves and be expressed, just as tears follow laughter and laughter follows tears.

This book contains all the best games, improvisations and dance structures I have found. I have not written about guided visualisation, art therapy or other therapeutic processes as there are many good books around on these subjects already. Play is the most neglected area of the Alternative/Human Potential/New Age Movement and this book is a small effort to change that. I hope you enjoy it and find it useful.

London, May 1994

Second Edition 2014

In 1987 I changed the basis of my work from the psychotherapy model to the shamanistic model, based on the ways of ancient cultures. This model beings together psychology, psychotherapy, hypnotherapy, spirituality and pretty much all healing and developmental modalities into one unified body of knowledge. I have been very much influenced by the teachings of the Medicine Wheel and found I was able to expand my work to address much more of the spiritual/psychological sicknesses of our time. I founded Eagle's Wing Centre for Contemporary Shamanism and incorporated Play-World and the work with play into a much wider body of work which could take people deeper and which incorporated many more tools and resources.

one
WHY PLAY?

'The young come into the Earth's system of life as if play were what they were created for.'

BRIAN SWIMME, *THE UNIVERSE IS A GREEN DRAGON*

The young of the higher mammals play. If you have ever had a kitten or a puppy, you will have seen them play, and very likely you played with them. This is a natural part of growing up, but it's not 'just play', it is an essential formative part of learning to be in a body. Learning helps the connecting of the neural networks which a human being needs in order to function. Play is both imaginative and logical and is material learning about what physically happens as a result of an action. Action and reaction, sense of balance and creativity, are all stimulated by play. If they are fun and we want to do them, then how much easier things seem and how much more pleasurable and rewarding is our life. Play can be formulated as a series of challenges from which a child – or adult – learns in a way that is positive and that brings self-esteem. When each step is 'winnable', and the competition is primarily with ourselves, we learn and gain in confidence. Play is brain training!

Teaching about Play for Adults

Accepting v. Blocking

Do you accept what life serves up, or do you block it? If an imaginary ball comes to you in a game, do you accept the proposition and play, letting your imagination have free reign, or do you block and hand the game on to the next person quickly? This tells a great deal about how heavily conditioned you are. When we block life, we tend to blame the situation or other people. The most heavily conditioned people who come to a play session rationalise their fear by finding it stupid so that they don't feel they have to take part! I remember one woman years ago who complained that the opening circle – a group of people standing in a circle holding hands – was too weird. For some, the journey to unlearn adulthood is a long one. Keith Johnstone, in his wonderful book *Impro* (2012), says he likes to think of normal adults as atrophied children! He says:

> Many 'well-adjusted' adults are bitter, uncreative, frightened, unimaginative and rather hostile people. Instead of assuming they were born that way, or that that's what being an adult entails, we might consider them as people damaged by their education and upbringing.
>
> (2012, p.78)

Trust

The second teaching is about trust. Trust in the moment, in the process of life itself and in yourself. I am not talking about naive trust in other humans but trust (faith) in life's process. Dare you improvise a role-play without any preconceived idea of what you are going to say and do? Any child could do that, and that means you could also do it when you were a child. Can you now? If not, what happened to stop you? How were you injured so that part of your nature got stuck? Can you become unstuck? Yes you can; by playing again and again until the old tapes in the mind are erased by new experience, allowing the old habituated fears to be experienced as unreal.

Surrender

The third teaching is about surrender. Surrender is trust taken to the next stage, accepting at the deepest level that the Universe is beneficent and loving, and choosing to co-operate with it. In surrendering to the spirit of the moment we become channels for the Life Force to move through us, rather than egos trying to be clever or funny. Once we have accepted the idea that we don't have to prove anything and we do what we do for the sake of doing it and for no ulterior motive, real play can happen.

The Two Tenets of Play-World

No 1: No Competition

No winners and no losers. Or no losers, so everybody is a winner.

The enemies to our happiness and joy in life are not outside ourselves but inside. The extremes of competition that many of us play out in sport, work, home, relationships and in other aspects of life, are a symptom of our lack of self-esteem. People who truly feel good about themselves do not need to prove that they can win. Competition can be a spur to greater achievement, but it also isolates people.

The cliché about loneliness at the top is a true one, and at the bottom of the ladder there tends to be resentment, anger and jealousy, all of which keep us separate from one another.

In this masculine-dominated, patriarchal society, we have lost the fullness of the feminine qualities. The qualities of the Mother – giving birth, making a home, growth, caring, nurturing, empathy, receptiveness, the ability to know and trust in the life process and the ability to use fully the inner self, the imagination. The imagination is the realm of the mage, the magician, the knowing that comes from a real connection to the deep, feminine, sub-conscious/unconscious. Instead, we have accepted the masculine idea that only that which is material or visible in the outer world is of value. Thus, half of our consciousness is denied its true place.

We can put this in another way and, looking at the Greek gods, say that we have elevated the god Apollo at the expense of the god Dionysus. We have raised up the masculine Apollonian qualities of light, truth, order and logic, and have suppressed the feminine Dionysian qualities of emotion, intuition and feeling. Dionysus has been relegated to the image of the goat, and orthodox religions have equated this energy, in their most out of touch moments, to the concept of the devil. As such, it comes out in wars and savagery, because it is an archetypal energy that must be expressed somehow. In this New Age of changing consciousness, the energy that is Dionysus is beginning once again to be honoured and expressed in healthier ways. Play is a Dionysian activity!

No 2: There Are No Mistakes –
Nothing Ever Goes Wrong!

There is an old saying which states that 'the person who never made a mistake never made anything'. The problem, however, is not making mistakes but *fear* of making mistakes. I see so many people missing out by not daring, not risking. We fear making a mistake, thinking we may look a fool to others. The fear is fear of being judged, and those who judge others first and foremost judge themselves. By creating an atmosphere where it really is OK to make mistakes, where there is no such thing as criticism, where no contribution is judged, where 'good' and 'bad' or 'success' and 'failure' are no longer criteria, where a game or structure that 'goes wrong' simply becomes a new game, we can come together without having to be on the defensive, and we can take the opportunity to *risk*, to be freely, impulsively and spontaneously creative. This is very different to most interactions in society; it is a big step for many people to be able to drop their defences and at first it can feel unfamiliar. There is a Medicine Wheel I learned from Cherokee-Metis Shaman Harley Swiftdeer called 'the mistakes wheel' and it looks like this:

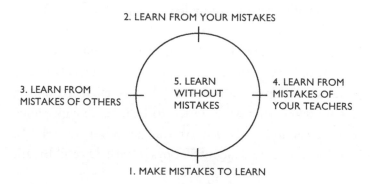

2. LEARN FROM YOUR MISTAKES

3. LEARN FROM
MISTAKES OF OTHERS

5. LEARN
WITHOUT
MISTAKES

4. LEARN FROM
MISTAKES OF
YOUR TEACHERS

1. MAKE MISTAKES TO LEARN

17

Mistakes are our way of learning; we humans seldom manage to learn without mistakes. The thing is to make different mistakes and not the same old ones over and over again! The person who can learn without making his own mistakes is an advanced one!

'The one thing one never regrets in life is one's mistakes.'

OSCAR WILDE

A Society Based on Competition

An overly competitive society inculcates self-doubt. If being OK depends on being a winner, then according to that society you are only OK so long as you are a winner. If you are anywhere else on the scale, you are a loser and so are not OK! If you are a winner, how long are you going to be able to maintain your place before someone beats you into second place and you become an ex-winner? There is no feeling of security in any of that; no chance to feel good about yourself for long, no possibility of real self-confidence, only the phoney kind – bravado – the false ego-self. If one is to be judged on extraneous factors such as results, class, possessions and rank, rather than as a person, how can one be expected to have anything like real self-confidence?

I was dispatched to boarding school at the age of eight, though it felt more like jail! At 13 I was sent to a senior jail, one of Great Britain's great 'public' (that actually means private and expensive) schools. Well, a fairly great one, at least that's what we were led to believe. Though public it most certainly was *not*! At this school there were 12 boarding houses with about 50 boys in each. Like all British education of the old-fashioned kind, the sexes were fully segregated until the age of 18 (puberty was to happen late by decree of the system). Between the 12 houses everything was competitive, even singing. Team spirit was all-important, and while that meant 'playing the game' in a fair way, it also meant *winning*! There was an unwritten law that a boy had no value whatsoever, except in what he could win for the school, his house or, lastly, himself. Lousy for your self-esteem if you dared to be merely average; catastrophic if you were not naturally good at sports like cricket or rugby, or had some special skill somewhere on the sports field or could shine in academia or some other field.

In no way is all competition bad; what is in question is the basis laid down by our society for the way we relate to one another. Competition, when it is the dominant way of relating, isolates and separates people. Not all societies have been based on such a degree of competition as ours and have created so much pain through separation and isolation. The living conditions of a separate society are the bed-sit, the one-parent family and the nuclear family. Tribal and village societies lived in much bigger units with all generations present and were based on co-operation, which they learned as children. Competition, when in the service of society and its individuals, is designed to spur us on to greater things. When we compete on the basis of mutual co-operation and support, society benefits, because the real basis of the relationship is co-operation and not competition. The problems start when it becomes more important to win than to play, and, sadly, that is how it is much of the time in the Western world today.

The Greatest Epidemic Sickness in Western Society

At the age of 18 I went into the car industry as a trainee. One of the first things that we were asked was, 'What is the purpose of the company?' The company was Rootes Group and it made cars and trucks, so we all came up with wonderful answers such as 'to make better cars', 'to make better value for money cars', 'to make longer lasting and more economical cars' and so on. None of us got the answer they wanted, which was, 'To make money!' The primary purpose of the company was its own survival and profit, not its service to the community. This was our first lesson in how to think like a man of industry and commerce.

The result of this way of thinking is the gross epidemic of personal self-doubt, lack of self-worth and, ultimately, of self-hatred and despair. This causes alienation of the individual, who feels that society is out to defeat him. This – not cancer, heart disease, AIDS, unemployment, etc. – is the real epidemic sickness in our society.

Education

The word 'education' comes from *'educare'* which means 'to bring out that which is within'. Much of our old-fashioned school education is about pumping in rather than bringing out; pumping in information, society's values and norms, the approved version of our history, the approved version of God and religion, and programming the child to learn lots and lots of facts – facts according to the thinking of the consensus. A yoga teacher from Liverpool called Ken Ratcliffe, from whom I learned a great deal in the

60s, referred to it as 'injurecation', combining the words 'education' and 'injury'. So much is aimed at developing the critical faculty to the detriment of intuition and inspiration. With an overdeveloped inner critic, one gets stuck in judgement and comparison. This issue was beautifully dramatised in the film *Dead Poets Society*, where the inspired teacher moved the students to creativity yet was finally dismissed for 'unusual teaching methods' and replaced by a typical, critically minded patriarch. Frequent disputes in British education between the government and much of the teaching profession cover this ground. I frequently wonder if anything is ever learned from the past.

Imagination Comes before Reality!

'Imagination is more important than knowledge.'

EINSTEIN

There is a dreadful saying, 'Oh, it's only imagination', often said to gifted children to reduce them to the state of lesser mortals. But it is based on a totally fallacious way of seeing the world, because imagination comes before reality. Look at the building you are in. Was it built before anyone thought of it? No, of course not! Someone thought of it – we could say 'dreamed it' – then probably an architect drew up plans and many other people added their ideas. Finally, the builders came in and actually placed the bricks and mortar. The very last thing that happened was the creation of 'reality'. It's the same with this book I am typing now. It started with a thought in my head – I 'dreamed it'! Now I am making it 'real' by typing it, then the editors will go through it and correct my grammar (I hope!) and finally it will go to the printers and become a book. But even then, when it is a 'real' book, what is its value? Its only value is in the ideas it conveys to you, the reader. Its value is entirely imaginal! Its value is in what it does for your imagination.

The Magical Child and the Wounded Child

'Save ye be as little children, ye shall not enter the Kingdom of Heaven.'

ST. MATTHEW, 18, VERSE 3

'A wise man is one who has not lost his child's heart.'

MENG TSE, ANCIENT CHINESE SAGE

'It is simpler to open the heart like a child than to unravel life's mysteries with thought.'

SRI CHINMOY, CONTEMPORARY SAGE

'We neglect our "child", but our child is the only living being in us.'

PROFESSOR ARNOLD KEYSERLING

'I feel God too – it's when I'm playing and I forget everything.'

RHEA, AGED 6

Sages throughout recorded history have spoken of 'the child within'. There are two children within each of us, the Magical Child and the Wounded Child; in the terms of Transactional Analysis, the Free Child and the Adapted

Child. Or we can call them the Innocent and the Orphan. It is the free – the magical/divine/innocent child – that we are seeking to release in the process of play. As we liberate the Magical Child, a time will come when the Wounded Child will show its face, when suppressed grief and rage will surface. This is natural and is discussed further in Chapter 2.

We can put these aspects of ourselves on the Medicine Wheel.

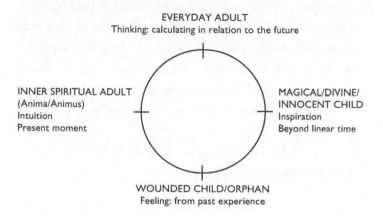

EVERYDAY ADULT
Thinking: calculating in relation to the future

INNER SPIRITUAL ADULT
(Anima/Animus)
Intuition
Present moment

MAGICAL/DIVINE/
INNOCENT CHILD
Inspiration
Beyond linear time

WOUNDED CHILD/ORPHAN
Feeling: from past experience

The Medicine Wheel is a wonderful guide to understanding ourselves. It is generally understood now in our society that disease is psychosomatic, that the mind influences the body. However, the Medicine Wheel teaches us that we have four aspects and we need to widen our perspective to include the emotions and the spirit. We are physical, emotional, mental and spiritual beings. I would like to put in here some background Medicine Wheel information which will help to convey a sense of this beautiful circular (and spiral) way of seeing and understanding the world in which we live, and will help explain some of the concepts which follow.

The Medicine Wheel

The Native American Medicine Wheel is a beautiful way of expressing teaching in a circular manner. All of life is in circles and spirals, even a straight line far enough out into the cosmos, we are assured by physicists, is curved, because space itself is curved. The Medicine Wheel teaches balance and harmony in all things, and shows us that we need always to look in four directions. We have four aspects: physical, mental, emotional and spiritual, just as there are four seasons and four sides to a square, four cardinal directions, four elements, four kingdoms and four primary sub-atomic forces.

Here is a wheel of the four primary elements of existence and the four aspects of ourselves.

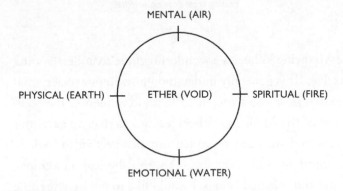

Each of our four aspects has a natural role to play.

The physical body holds and contains us, not in any restrictive sense, but just like a jar holds jam, it holds together all that we are.

The emotions are for feeling and expressing (i.e. 'giving'). When we express clearly and cleanly how we feel, we communicate our truth. When emotions get dammed up, as for example in the tradition of the stiff upper lip, we learn how to hold emotions in instead of expressing them and, if pushed too far, tend to 'give' with the body instead, for example in an expression of violence.

The mind is for receiving and sifting information, for sorting truth from falsity and wisdom from 'bullshit'. The mind is the intellect and a good intellect helps us to steer our way through life's journey.

The spirit, our inner essence, is for determining, choosing and directing our path, our life journey. There is an old saying, 'Make up your mind!' Instead, how about using your mind to sort and sift like a computer, but when it comes to decisions to sense into your inner essence, to let spirit influence you. Now we can add these to the wheel.

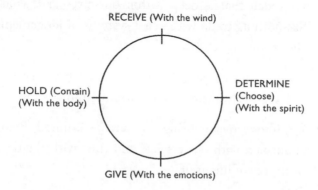

Each of the four directions has an 'ally' and these four 'allies' make for balance in life. By developing these qualities we bring harmony and balance into ourselves.

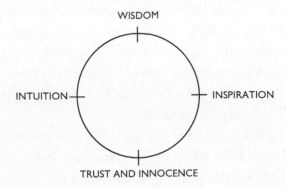

- *Trust* means trust in the Universe, in the process of life itself. It does not mean naive trust in other people. *Innocence* means inner sense, not naiveté, being 'in your essence', in your centre.

- *Wisdom* means inner knowing. It is the knowledge we touch that is deep within ourselves and which has nothing to do with belief systems or judgements about things.

- *Intuition* means listening to our inner knowing and hearing the 'still small voice' from within.

- *Inspiration* means being 'in-spirit' – inspired. Being connected with our essence and thus with the deep processes of life itself.

The Medicine Wheel is a multi-layered way of seeing the world and the forces that act upon us and within the cosmos. The wheels previously mentioned are just a minute fraction of the teaching.

Once one understands the essence of the Medicine Wheel, life becomes much more comprehensible. These teachings are one of the greatest gifts I have received in my life.

Play and Humour Are Not Always a Funny Business!

I need to make some uncomfortable points. The joys of childhood play are only one side of the coin. What about the cruelty that sometimes arises? What about the exclusion of one seen to be different, the familiar cry of 'You're out', the scapegoating, the exclusion from the pack, the bullying of the physically weaker and often more sensitive by the stronger and often less sensitive kids?

A society which teaches children competition as the way of learning encourages all those negative emotions, as it teaches that everyone who is not a winner is a loser and inadequate. In a class of say 20 – or however big it is – there can only be one who comes top. Everyone else is thus taught that they are lesser. There is a fascinating story about children in the Peruvian Andes being taught football by the conquering Europeans a couple of centuries ago. The children really liked football and got to play it regularly. Then the Europeans noticed something odd. Their game ended when the scores were equal. Apparently it took about a year to teach the children that there must be a winning team and a losing team!

In the realm of humour too, there is that which enlightens and that which endarkens. There is the humour which throws light on the human condition and the humour which simply stereotypes, judges, criticises and encourages prejudice. Let me list the qualities which seem to me to make the difference:

Enlightening Humour	Endarkening Humour
Creative	Destructive
Life enhancing	Life negating
Life observing	Life pre-judging
Aiding seeing and understanding	Aiding blindness
Accepting own foibles and imperfections	Knows better, in the right
Bringing closer together	Separating and dividing
Laughing with	Laughing at
Laughing at self	Laughing only at others
Caring and empathising	Contemptuous/insensitive
Allowing change	Promoting stuckness
Dialogues with the unknown	Rejecting the unknown

The cruel aspects of play and humour happen when the ego takes over and winning becomes all-important. Winning is about control. When to win is more important than to play, we enter the realm of the fascist, the control freak, the totalitarian.

Fascists don't laugh and play! Whatever humour they may enjoy will come into the destructive category, laughing at the misfortunes of others. Fascists are people who are very afraid of life yet are even more afraid to admit to their fear. Any one of us can become a fascist if we let fear take over and we don't face ourselves in the mirror of life. Fascists are what we become when we are so afraid that we want everything and everybody under control. The essence of play is that it is not under control, yet paradoxically it needs rules. It is chaos, yet it is chaos within a framework. A game requires agreements between the participants – rules – as a container within which chaos can reign safely for an agreed amount of time and within an agreed space. Yet these rules are also an agreed setting aside of normal rules; just as we set aside conventional rules, roles and expectations when we go to the theatre or movies. A session of creative play is a period of self-generated theatre in which the script is written in the moment. I see play as a dialogue with the unknown. If you know the outcome, it is no longer play. The more one tries to control the outcome, the less playful the activity becomes. The essence of play is spontaneity, 'nowness', presence; the first enemy of play is fear and inhibition.

There are two primary kinds of fear, which we can call 'real fear' and 'unreal fear'. 'Real fear' means what we feel in a life-threatening situation such as an earthquake, an accident, or a large vehicle descending rapidly upon us when we are standing in the middle of the road. We feel this at the back of the neck. We move – or our being moves itself – instantly, in the moment, totally devoid of self-importance, caring not a jot what anyone might think of us. Our being acts in the instant, with power. This kind of experience happens to most of us comparatively rarely and this fear is essential to our physical survival. But what of all the other bits and pieces of fear, shyness, anxiety, inhibition and worry that we feel about people and situations that are not life-threatening? This is what the term 'unreal fear' means, and we usually feel that in the solar plexus area. We are not life-threatened, yet we can feel sickeningly inhibited at times, like an actor having first-night nerves. All this kind of fear is rooted in our experience of the past and is about 'insuring' our future, it is not about the present at all! Our existence is not threatened, only our self-importance. The fear is that our mask might slip and we might become vulnerable and the pieces of ourselves we prefer to hide might become visible. We might lose our cool and let others see us 'naked', as we really are. Well, play and games as described in this book are about helping us to lose 'unreal fear' and become maskless. The Medicine Wheel way of saying it is to 'erase personal history', meaning to erase the negative effect of past traumas upon our present.

I have done an exercise with many workshop groups to elicit participants' personal negative mythology. The results read like this:

- I'm not good enough (this underlies the majority of personal mythologies).

- I'm unworthy.

- I'm unlovable. I'm not worthy enough to be in a loving relationship.

- I feel incapable. To want a relationship means I'm weak.

- I don't deserve, so I feel guilty when I receive.

- I fear failure. I fear success.

- I need your approval. The only way I can get approval is by hiding my true self.

- I fear taking my power. Others will reject me if I do.

- If I show my sexual feelings I won't be able to control what happens next.

- If I show who I really am, I will be abandoned and rejected.

- Unless I am powerless yet successful as a woman, my Dad won't love me.

- I make myself so independent no one can reject me.

- Because I don't let myself know what I want, I don't run the risk of getting it.

- I can't win!

- I am more spiritually evolved so you won't understand me.

- All-out attack is the best form of defence.

- Everyone else can do it; they're all bastards anyway.

- I'm misunderstood and superior.

I stress that these are the inner dialogues of generally well-adjusted people; people who know enough to seek quality in their lives. Yet this panoply of beliefs gives rise to their inner demons. Read through and see which ones mean something to you. This is the archetypal inner dialogue of the people of our culture. If you read it through all together as if one person is speaking, you have an archetype of the inner dialogue of a typical everyday nice, normal, ordinary neurotic.

The problem with beliefs is that what we believe deep inside tends to manifest. In the words of Henry Ford, 'Whether you think you can, or whether you think you can't, you're right!' To grow and flourish in life, each of us has to get to the core of our deeply held sub-conscious inner beliefs and change the ones that don't work for us.

Our society has come to be the way it is through the 'epidemic' I talked about earlier – the teaching through religion, education and upbringing of deep feelings of personal inadequacy, shame and guilt. The motivation to 'prove oneself', so overtly put to young men, and often more covertly to young women, is dependent on these feelings. If you feel adequate, what is there to prove? There are many stories about white people conquering indigenous tribal people around the world and attempting to set them to work like good Protestants. It never worked, and the tribal people were called lazy and indolent, but from their perspective work and acquisition are not the purpose of life. They hadn't been taught to think badly enough of themselves to be motivated to acquire wealth! They felt OK with a bare minimum, what we might think of as a life at subsistence level.

Feelings of inadequacy are the key to controllability. Carrot and stick. The powers that be hold the stick: if you do as you are told, maybe you will finally be permitted to feel OK about yourself by the time you collect your pension (if some enterprising entrepreneur or government hasn't stolen it!). The idea that a lousy life on Earth will be rewarded in Heaven after death is the grossest of manipulations and was used at the time of the Industrial Revolution (and so many other times) to con people into a life of virtual slavery.

There is a teaching called 'the Four Enemies of a Person of Knowledge' and it comes from Carlos Castaneda's *The Teachings of Don Juan*. I can represent it on a Medicine Wheel like this:

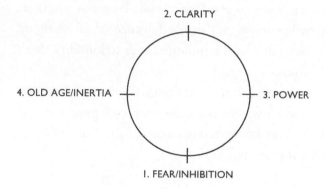

Fear/Inhibition

Play is a great way of confronting and losing fear.

The first 'enemy' is (unreal) fear, and it literally stops us being ourselves. Fear, inhibition, shyness, anxiety, worry, doubt – all these come between us and prevent us from expressing who we are. This is the opposite of 'trust' on the wheel of attributes I discussed earlier.

Clarity (I prefer to call it bullshit)

Play helps us to be open and not get stuck in clarity and dogma.

Know it all, got it right, I know best, mine is the right way, this is what you should do/could do/could have done, this is the way I do it.

'Oh no you shouldn't do it like that, you should do it like this', says Harry Enfield's wonderful Dad character, a marvellous archetype of the enemy of 'clarity'.

Good humour does battle with clarity. Knocking down the know-all is always good for a laugh. Bombast, pretence, pomposity, hypocrisy and ego-indulgence of all sorts are game for humour. Good humour leads us to humility, that's the real point.

It is great to feel clear about things. Clarity only becomes an 'enemy' when we get stuck and stop changing with the flow of life and become dogmatic (hence 'bullshit'). All dogma is atrophied wisdom.

Power

Play helps us to let go of attempts to control and have power over the situation and the actions of others.

Stop all this messing around. You take your orders from me. Come on, stop all that play nonsense, we are here for serious business, we are going to do things properly now...

Real power, power over oneself and one's life, comes with a sense of illumination and is a great attribute. After all, self-empowerment is what we seek and is the essence of much of the teaching in this book. The problem, however, is summed up in the saying 'Absolute power corrupts absolutely'. I would add 'Absolute powerlessness also corrupts absolutely'. It is very difficult to control ourselves when we hold vast power and to use it only for good. It is also difficult to guide ourselves creatively through life when we feel utterly powerless. The key is to seek power within, over the many aspects of our self.

There is a lovely chant which says:

'Freedom, we can have our freedom, freedom, we can have our freedom,
Freedom comes from not hangin' on, you've got to let go, let go, let go!'

Interestingly the original words I was taught for the first line were 'Freedom, won't you give us freedom', but who can give us freedom? If it takes someone else to give me freedom, then I am dependent on that person and am not free (not at all free!).

Old Age/Inertia

Play helps us to defeat inertia and stay young, whatever physical age we may be.

Too tired, too old, can't be bothered, why try to change things anyway? Everything is good enough the way it is. We're all going to die anyway so why bother, stop rocking the boat. Let's keep it all safe – the way it used to be. Put the kettle on and let's have a nice cup of tea.

To quote the comedian George Burns, 'You can't stop getting older but you can stop getting old'. Old age comes to all of us naturally but there are many ways of growing old. I am talking here about inertia – premature ageing, loss of intuition, loss of spirit. There is nothing old about the 100-year-old Native Americans I have met except their bodies, and even then they are incredibly fit compared with most of us.

Let us look at the process of getting into the spirit of play and dance, and in fact any activity in which we wish to involve ourselves deeply. We can put that process on a Medicine Wheel like this:

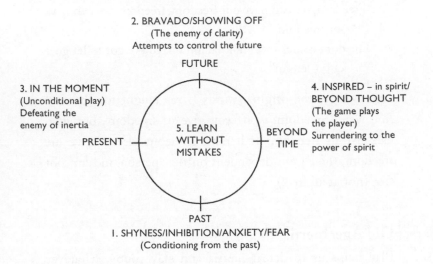

2. BRAVADO/SHOWING OFF
(The enemy of clarity)
Attempts to control the future

FUTURE

3. IN THE MOMENT
(Unconditional play)
Defeating the
enemy of inertia

PRESENT

5. LEARN
WITHOUT
MISTAKES

BEYOND
TIME

4. INSPIRED – in spirit/
BEYOND THOUGHT
(The game plays
the player)
Surrendering to the
power of spirit

PAST
1. SHYNESS/INHIBITION/ANXIETY/FEAR
(Conditioning from the past)

When people come together in any setting, there is a measure of shyness, inhibition and anxiety, 'unreal fear', as discussed earlier. Then some of us tend to move into bravado – that feeling of overcoming fear, yet actually still being afraid. It takes time to get out of the conditioning of the past and anxiety about the future and to get into the present, and thus be in the moment and in a place of full authenticity.

It is interesting to ponder that full authenticity happens when we are not trying to be anything special at all, but simply 'beingness' is expressing itself through us. When I am not trying to be 'me', I can be authentically me! Happiness can then happen within me, creativity can occur through me, authentic expression can occur as me… But then, who am 'I'? I am an open channel for *Life Force* to express itself! I become inspired, 'in-spirit'. I can live in a state of happiness and joy, devoid of self-doubt, self-criticism, self-denigration and so on. All those old demons lie down and become allies and friends. That's bliss!

Unconditional Love

Non-competitive play is a great way to re-learn a co-operative and loving way of relating. Loving in a non-sexual, non-specific, unconditional way, as meant by the Greek word 'agape'. In our language we have only one word for love – a serious oversight leading to much confusion. Love is continually confused with sex and partnering, so much so that agape has been largely lost as a concept. We can translate agape as lovingness – living in a state of lovingness towards all creation. The feeling is not conditional upon what happens outside. We no longer say 'I love you and you alone' or 'I love you for what you do for me'. Unconditional love exists regardless of an object because it is an internal state of being, a state of being in lovingness within oneself. From a state of lovingness within, one is then naturally in unconditional lovingness with all that is without. This is the basis of community. We are all on a journey somewhere and we all help each other to get there. This is co-operative team spirit.

Playing with people in a non-competitive way engenders unconditional lovingness. Through games and role-playing we get to show something of ourselves, to drop pieces of our mask and let our vulnerability show. When we see one another's vulnerability – when we see the truth of each other – we recognise our oneness and we can dare to love one another, to be in a state of lovingness with one another unconditionally and without expectation. Then we can dare to put ourselves in front of people and risk failure – or success – and whatever happens, it will be OK.

In my travels I picked up an anonymous poem relating to this subject.

Risk

To laugh is to risk appearing the fool,
To weep is to risk appearing sentimental,
To reach out for another is to risk involvement,
To expose feelings is to risk exposing your true self,
To place your ideas, your dreams before the crowd is to
    risk their loss,
To love is to risk not being loved in return,
To live is to risk dying,
To hope is to risk despair,
To try is to risk failure.
But risks must be taken, because the greatest hazard in
    life is to risk nothing.
The person who risks nothing, does nothing, has nothing
    and is nothing…
He simply cannot learn, feel, change, grow, love, and live.
Chained by his certitudes, he is a slave.
He has forfeited his freedom.
Only a person who risks is free.

                            William Arthur Ward

Happiness

Happiness is something you know you have just had!

The problem with happiness is that the more you seek it, the more elusive it becomes. The more you try to achieve it, the more the judgemental mind compares, questions, criticises and doubts – and happiness is gone. Furthermore, the moment we know we have it, it tends to mysteriously disappear – or at least the fullness of it does, the magical quality. It is when we are 'lost' in that which makes us happy that we have real happiness. Putting that in the form of a Zen Koan:

'When happiness is, I am not!'

Most of us can remember times in childhood when we were totally absorbed in play, or rather we can remember the moments just afterwards – such as when a parent called us to bed and we found there had been a kind of time-warp. What felt to us like minutes was actually several hours, hours of glorious, total absorption. We were 'lost' in joyful activity. These are the real moments of happiness, so is it any wonder we cannot find them when we search for them?

Happiness is a by-product of involvement, absorption, intent, focus. It is not something to seek for its own sake, as the mere effort of seeking it keeps it away. In interaction games, dance and theatre improvisation, you can find ways through which happiness can come as a result of losing your little ego-self, so that the Magical Child self can materialise through you. The object of the games and structures in this book is to help you to 'lose yourself to find yourself'; to achieve a state of ecstasy. Once you develop the ability to enter the Magical Child space easily, it is then possible to maintain the state of happiness while being conscious of it. This is how the observer – consciousness – develops.

Play allows us expression of our true self without regard for the rules of 'normal life', and in so doing it allows us to see more of who we really are and who we might become.

A Native American sculpting a piece of wood considers him/herself a tool of the Creator in releasing the carving that is already there, obscured by the wood around it. A Westerner, imbued with our ego-centred culture, would consider himself a great (or not so great) sculptor and judge himself by the results. Thus the Westerner's self-concept is dependent upon the view of others in the external world; the Native American's on his own inner view. What a difference that makes!

'All deeds which do not flow from your Inner Self are dead before God.'

MEISTER ECKHART

two

A GUIDE TO BEING
A FACILITATOR

A facilitator is someone who 'makes it easy'! To work with these games means to be in the spirit of these games yourself, that is to be spontaneous, non-judgemental, trusting and unconditionally loving towards the inner beings of all who come to play with you. It doesn't matter if you happen not to like the personality of any of your participants, you can still be loving towards their essence.

Be aware of the group energy; how it is in the beginning and how it fluctuates during the activity. If a game goes well and most players are 'with it', let it run. If a game isn't working well, cut it short and go on to something else. If the energy is high, go with a series of high energy games and then, when you sense the group is ready, change to an introspective, gentle structure such as a trust game, Car Wash or the Mirror Dance. If the energy is low, don't fight it, go with it and change your programme accordingly. The chances are that the energy will spontaneously rise later on, as low energy is usually motivated by fear, and if you proceed gently and slowly, the fear will begin to evaporate.

One tenet that is most important: *The participants are never wrong!*

If they do something different from what you asked them, if there is a fault to be found, it is with you. At no time whatever should you show even a hint of judgement or negativity towards them. You are asking them to be open and vulnerable, you are the 'parent' for the session. Whatever you do, don't behave like one! Your task is to give them what a good parent would have given them when they were a child – unconditional love and acceptance. The chances that this is what they got in their childhood living in the 'developed' world are remote, sadly. Robert Bly, the American poet, jokes that the proportion of dysfunctional families in the USA is 102 per cent. Well, in Britain I reckon it's only 101 per cent (or maybe even less!) but it is still a high percentage. The majority of 'normal' families are dysfunctional to some degree. Your task as a leader is to give people a taste of something different. That is how you will make magic. Once they realise that you are totally non-threatening and you are there for them, they will trust you and let you lead them into all sorts of experiences in which they are actually very vulnerable. In doing this you help to give them back lost portions of themselves. You help them to retrieve pieces of themselves they had to repress in order to survive as a child.

There is a natural wave-form to a workshop, like the sine wave. It is most clearly seen in a five-day, or longer, workshop. The group comes together, plays together, people meet each other and enjoy each other; energy is high. This is the honeymoon period! Then the irritations begin to surface, people's defences become visible, their self-limitations show – the person who hides grief under a fixed smile, the one whose constant jokes become unfunny. The people are ready to plumb the depths, and this must be helped to happen. There must be space and help for all who need to explore the darkness. Then there is the time when, just as the laughter turns to tears, so the tears turn back to laughter and the group is ready to play again, only this time at a new and much deeper level. This is where the 'gold' is. Barriers are down, fear and shyness have gone, there is no longer a need to defend or show off, we can be together in the moment, spontaneous, naturally creative, flowing, easy, relaxed.

The psychologist Bruce Tuckman coined a neat way of describing the archetypal group process:

Forming/norming/storming/performing/adjourning – mourning.

A group comes together, it is formed and the members skirt around each other, attracted by some and repelled by others. Then there is the honeymoon period – the 'falling-in-love' period – 'norming', the being-nice-to-everyone period. Then the storm clouds gather and blunt truths get spoken. The chips are down, feathers fly and everybody's projections get an airing. After that is the time when the group can really work together creatively and intuitively, as the illusions have gone, the members see each other warts and all, and accept each other for who and what they are and can then really help each other to manifest the best of each other. This is the time of real love as against 'falling-in-love'. Finally comes the parting time, the time of good-bye, of mourning.

When facilitating a workshop longer than a day, it is most likely that you will encounter the Wounded Child in some of your participants. Some of them will laugh till they cry. I said earlier that it is necessary to have therapy skills, but if you are not a therapist and emotions come up, don't try to know best. The fundamental skill is not to try to be clever, not to panic, just to remember that your client's body knows and will give you cues as to what they need. You are there to support the client just as you are in the games, dancing and improvisations. Sometimes they just need to cry and be supported. Sometimes people need to express anger and need your support and permission to do so, and a cushion or two so they can express it safely. When this happens, you can be sure that group sharing time will be needed afterwards to help participants to ground themselves and bring themselves back to equilibrium. If a lot has happened, you can invite them to find a partner and share in twos or threes, and then bring the whole circle together to share.

Sharing Circles

When sharing, a good way to ensure that everyone has a chance to be heard is to pass an object around the circle, such as a 'talking-stick' or stone. Whoever holds the object takes their turn to speak and to be heard until they choose to pass the stick on. This avoids the problem of people competing for time and others getting agitated because they fear they will never get their moment. Adjust the size of the sharing circles according to the time available. If there is time and there are not too many people, it is good to hear a whole group; if not maybe groups of three/four/five would be appropriate. With reflective issues and not much time, pairs are best.

Props

- A good and varied selection of recorded music (see Resources for suggestions).

- Hats and scarves. A collection of old hats and scarves, bits of material, and so on is a wonderful help to participants to get into role-play. Oxfam and similar charity shops are good sources.

- Paper and crayons, Blu-tack, etc. I have not written about the use of drawing, art therapy and guided visualisation in this book, as there are many good books on those subjects, but it is very handy to have materials available.

- A cushion or two.

- Candles and tray or holder, for quiet moments, chanting/singing with lights dimmed.

- Drum and/or rattle. Helpful when leading chants or songs.

- Unusual objects for 'One Minute Please' commercials/ theatre pieces, etc.

- Bell, whistle, clanger – a selection of attention-getting devices for you to maintain a measure of control!

- 'Talking-stick' or stone for sharing circles.

three
WARM UP GAMES

Starting a Session

Starting a session is very important because it sets the tone for everything to follow. Gather everyone together in a circle – a circle is a symbol of equality and is the least hierarchical of structures into which to welcome everyone.

'Well, hello everybody, welcome to Play-World. Tonight there is an open space, and some recorded music, but no TV, no movies, no experts, just us!'

Introduce yourself and the purpose of this time to be spent together. When the group are mainly strangers to each other, and when they are unfamiliar with this kind of activity, it is most important to start in a way which is as unthreatening as possible.

Get them to breathe deeply, stretch the body and then make sounds.

A good exercise at this point is:

Dump the 'Shit'

This exercise encourages participants to dump the 'shit' (or 'stuff' or 'angst' if you prefer politeness!) of the day.

Breathe deeply and throw the angst of the day, whatever you wish to let go of, into the middle of the circle with a big sound.

This always gets energy moving and also gives you a feeling for the mood of the group. It is also like exorcising whatever concerns or anxieties the people are carrying from the outside world so that they, and you, can all 'be here now'.

Now continue the process.

Rag Doll

Shake loose various parts of the body; hands, arms, feet, legs and whole body as if it were a rag doll; and while you are doing this, mumble!

Another way to continue warming up is:

Funniest Joke

Imagine someone has just told the funniest joke in the universe and let yourself laugh (20–30 seconds maximum).

A good follow-on exercise I have often used to get people feeling more present and ready to play is:

Italian Breathing

Imagine you are an Italian – naturally you express everything with your hands. Take three deep breaths and use your arms to bring the breath to you. Then crouch down. Breathe in while coming up to standing, lift your arms above your head, stretch and complete the inbreath. Exhale and gradually sink back down to crouching. Repeat this sequence two or three times.

Then, standing, breathe in like an Italian with all the help you can get from your arms; look at someone across the circle and on the outbreath throw a sound across to them.

This gets people properly aerated and the last part generates interaction and usually some laughter and relaxation.

Spiral

Start with a standing circle, holding hands. You can use recorded music of your choice, but a very nice way to do this is to get everyone singing a simple song or chant. For example, a Native American chant like this:

'Earth my body, water my blood,
Air my breath and fire my spirit.'

Or this Arapaho Ghost Dance song:

'I circle around, I circle around, the boundaries of the earth, wearing my long wing feathers as I fly.'

(Both these chants can be learned from the tape and booklet I made with a group of friends – *Forty-Four Chants – Words and Music* [see Resources]. They are very easy to learn and to teach, as people can pick them up in a few moments.)

When you have got the chant going, let go with your right hand and lead the circle to your right, with everyone following you, into a spiral formation winding inward. As you come into the centre and when the circle is tightening into a spiral but not too tight, turn sharply and then wind around the opposite way, reversing direction. When you are back on the outside, reverse direction again and then wind the circle back into a spiral, finishing when the circle is as tight as is comfortable (see diagram).

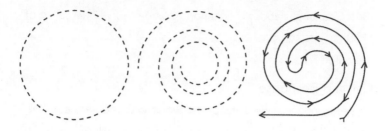

Before you start, invite everyone as they spiral around to 'see' the other people they are about to spend time with, and to let themselves 'be seen'. This formation movement enables everyone to make a connection with everyone else.

Moving Circle

This is another nice and very simple way to achieve the same feeling of meeting:

Everyone stands in a circle, holding hands. Put on some nice music of your choice. Holding with both hands, move in towards the people opposite, gently pulling the people either side of you. Then pull out, and then in and out and so on until the circle moves in and out and around on its own and all sorts of things happen spontaneously.

Chants

Put a candle in the centre and invite everyone to sit around in a circle.

Singing chants together is very beautiful and evocative. Simple well-known songs such as 'Michael Row the Boat' or 'Kumbaya' or 'Row, Row, Row Your Boat' are also really chants in that they convey a feeling and are simple, repetitive and easy to learn. Chanting is not music *per se* and is not about singing 'well' or in tune. Chanting is about meditation, it's about a feeling, a sense of togetherness and oneness.

Call and Response

The Ancients in many parts of the world would ease their work by chanting. One person would 'call' a simple melody, usually in eight beats, 'Hey heyo ya ho' and the others would answer like an echo, 'Hey heyo ya ho'. The words and melody of the call vary and it works well to invite all who wish to take a turn at calling. This is a great way to get a group's energy moving.

A variation on that is:

Hoeing or Digging

Get everyone in the circle to turn to the right (only because most are right handed) and start to mime hoeing the ground. Then start the call and response.

Having got everyone breathing, feeling relaxed, at ease and comfortable about being there, the next stage is to get them meeting each other and interacting.

Name Games

Name games are necessary warmers unless you opt for name tags. Personally I dislike being 'labelled', but it does serve its purpose if you have a group of more than 40. Here are some games to avoid tags. My favourite is the first one.

Whisper Name Game

Ask participants to mill around and make contact; each person is to whisper their *own* name in the ears of the others.

After a minute or two ring a bell, bang a gong, clap or what you will – to get everyone's attention. Ask them to continue mingling and as they meet someone to whisper the *other person's* name in that person's ear! Tell them if they forget just to make a guess – their partner will correct them if necessary.

This causes great hilarity as people try to remember each other's name. By the end of the game they are likely to remember quite a few!

Name Cushion

You need a cushion for this one!

In a standing circle, throw a cushion to someone and say your name.

When most folks have learnt enough names, change the rules to: 'Throw the cushion to someone and say their name as you throw.'

Name Crescendo

In a standing circle, all together crouch down low and whisper your name, getting louder as you gradually stand up and go on tiptoe. After the crescendo, get smaller and quieter as you go down to crouch and whisper. Then one person at a time states his name and leads the group in a crescendo of his name.

Name Echo

In a standing circle, one person says his name with any sound and action.

The group echoes this twice. Everyone takes a turn, going round the circle.

Alternatively, each participant comes into the centre of the circle for his turn.

A hilarious variation is for the whole process to slowly speed up.

Terrific Teresa

Again the group is in a standing circle. Take turns to introduce yourselves by adding a word before your name, beginning with the same letter. It works well to enact the character suggested in the words: *Jumping Jeremy/Lascivious Liz/Gorgeous George.*

On paper, this kind of game looks unbelievably corny. Whether it is in practice or not depends on the spirit of the moment. It can be hilarious when entered into fully and played to the hilt, but completely destroyed by cynicism. Cynicism is a destroyer not only of play but of love and all tender emotions.

Fantasy Names and Introductions

Get everyone to partner up and spend a minute or two to think of a fantasy self and tell this to your partner. Back in the circle, your partner will then introduce this fantasy you, and in turn you introduce his own fantasy self.

For example: 'Introducing Peerless Pete the Aviator, just back from navigating the globe' (Pete 'flies' into the circle).

'Ladies and gentlemen, we are honoured to be in the presence this evening of Big Mac, the belly dancer from Brighton.' (I can't imagine what kind of action that would lead to!)

'I am delighted to introduce Dame Edna Beverage, the tea lady from Ruislip.' (Edna mimes offering tea and whatever around the circle.)

Movement and Sound Games

These games take place in a standing circle. They are simple, mainly repetitive in structure and allow for endless creativity and spontaneity.

Movement Crescendo

This is a game which can be played with any number from about 6 to 40, even more if the leader has a loud voice!

The group is in a standing circle. The leader starts a simple movement and sound – small and quiet.

The group mirrors the leader, who then makes the movement and sound bigger and louder, and begins to move towards the centre.

The group follows, and everyone simultaneously moves forward until it builds to a crescendo. Everyone moves out again and the activity gets smaller and quieter until it fades away. Another member of the group starts another movement and sound, and so on.

VARIATION

It can become hilarious when words take over from sounds.

For example, 'This is ridiculous' or "Ello, 'ello, what's going on 'ere then?' or 'Shhh, be quiet' – which then inevitably ends up being shouted loudly!

This game is about letting go and being leader as well as follower. It is good for several people to take a turn at leading and in particular it is very good for shy people to lead. Also, it is good to encourage people to let a movement and sound 'come through them', not to think intellectually about what to do and so get stuck in trying to 'get it right'.

Sound and Movement Round

The leader creates a quick and simple sound and movement and passes it to the next person, who passes it on and so on around the circle.

VARIATIONS

1. The same sound and movement is passed around, e.g. the sound 'huh' together with a movement.

2. The movement and sound can change as it goes around.

3. The movement and sound does change with each person.

4. Pass the same movement and sound onwards, or a different one backwards around the circle.

This is a good opener. Simple and quick, it raises energy without taxing either shyness or improv skills, and lets those who are shy pass it on quickly, while those who aren't shy may enjoy a few moments of creativity (and those who like to show off have an opportunity to do so!).

Hot Coals

The leader begins playing with imaginary hot coals and it soon becomes clear what they are. Then she passes the hot coals on to the next player in the circle, who receives them and plays with them until they become something else (or stay hot coals) and so on around the circle. Alternatively, they can be passed across or to anyone in the circle.

Pass the Clap

The leader starts a clap, the next person claps and so on round the circle, getting faster and faster until it becomes one long clap.

Or, it goes quickly round but can reverse direction.

Or, it can change on reversing direction to a double clap – or treble clap – and so on.

From here on it's easy to add your own variations:

Face Pass

The leader makes a face and passes it to the next person in the circle.

This person has the choice to pass the same face (or as near as reasonably possible) to the next person in line, or to pass a different face backwards around the circle. And so on.

VARIATION

As soon as the simple structure is understood, add sound to go with the face.

This is a good game for helping people lose a few years and remember childhood. It is also good for losing inhibitions, because it's difficult to keep one's cool in a daft game like this! Also, it works very well in reconnecting people to the child within. I have found it dissolves resistance in some people who were not moved by other games.

Devils into Angels

This is really a variation on the last game.

The first person in the circle makes a devil-like pose, then turns to one side and faces the next person, who copies the pose and changes it into an angelic pose. He turns to the next person, who copies and changes into a devil and so on.

Imaginary Ball Toss

The leader has an imaginary ball which has size and weight.

The leader throws the 'ball' to another member of the circle, who catches it (probably).

The ball may change shape; for example, it may become a cat when gently handed to the next person, become a biting monster, become a giant when thrown across the circle and then a ladder up which the person mimes climbing and so on.

This is a very simple game but great fun when people let themselves go and the ball begins to change into all sorts of surprising things. I have been amazed at some of the weird things the ball has changed into and some of the wonderful lateral thinking that has come out of it. I tend to let this game go on for quite a long time when it takes off.

Changing Movements

One person goes into the middle and creates a movement with a sound.

He moves around exploring this movement and sound until it feels complete (from ten seconds up to a minute) and then takes it to someone else in the circle who copies it and moves into the centre, while the first person replaces the other in the circle.

The new person then explores the sound and movement, and lets it change organically into a creation of his own and then takes it to another member of the circle – and so on.

The important thing here is to let the sound and movement change organically without the intellect getting in the way.

Humming Circle

The leader hums a note, which the group copies. The leader then starts to hum an improvisation around the note.

When the leader feels she has expressed enough, it is passed to the next person, who becomes the improviser. And so on around the circle.

Orchestra and Conductor

Last, here is a collective game using sound. I was about to write 'music' but I don't remember the game ever quite making it into that exalted realm!

Warm the group up by getting them to hum, and make all sorts of vocal noises.

The group is the orchestra. Arrange them like an orchestra with small groups who contribute certain sounds, and then invite one member to come out front to be the conductor. He then conducts with arms all over the place trying to get some musical order out of what is usually a glorious racket!

This game works best when it is actually a bit orchestrated and organised.

Simple, Quick Warm Ups

Sound Game

The group hums a low note, then intones 'Aah…' and makes the lowest possible sound.

Then everyone makes the sound 'Eeeeee…' on the highest possible note.

Then everyone finds a partner, crouches down, holds his partner's hands and looks him in the eye.

They begin sounding the low note, and as they rise to standing on their toes, so the note rises up to the highest pitch and then it and they sink down again to the lowest.

All find another partner and repeat.

Wrong Names (from *Impro* by Keith Johnstone)

Everyone goes around the room very quickly and loudly gives the wrong names to 12 objects.

It's amazing how difficult this is. Our minds are so blocked with logical thinking that it takes a lot of practise for most people to free themselves and do this simple exercise easily.

Opposite Emotions (from *Playfair* by Matt Weinstein)

Get everyone to leap about with joy and shout, '*I'm depressed!*' (This is fundamentally impossible and causes hilarity.)

It can be followed with everyone getting into a thoroughly miserable pose and saying, '*I'm really happy*' ('I'm so happy I think I'll kill myself').

And then in a placating pose, '*I'm really very angry*', said very politely and nicely.

Then angrily, '*I love you*'.

And in a pleading, needy way, '*I really feel OK about myself*',('I really want you to know that!').

And so on, portraying the opposite emotion to that of the words.

From time to time, we all express the opposite with our words and deeds, so when we do it in a game, we also recognise something about ourselves and can laugh about it.

Physical Circle Games
Knot
Everybody comes together in the centre of the room, closes their eyes, reaches out their hands and clasps another hand.

When everyone is bonded hand to hand, it is time to open eyes and set about undoing the knot!

This involves a pleasing degree of chaos, stepping over and under, through and around until, with luck, the knot is untied.

When playing this game it is good to take it only as far as it goes easily. Sometimes the knot comes untied quite naturally and sometimes it doesn't. It is important not to be concerned about 'success'.

Lap Sit
Everybody stands in a circle. The group turns sideways and bunches up very close together, then gradually sits down. Hopefully, the knees of the person behind will become the seat of the one in front.

This is a good game for moving a shy kind of group towards greater intimacy, particularly if the circle collapses once or twice and people end up in a heap (which usually happens without any help!).

Shoulder Massage

Get everyone in the circle to turn to the right and then give a shoulder massage to the person in front. After a minute or so, all turn around and give massages the other way.

Partnered Line Games

I call these line games because I find they work best with everyone in two lines, each participant facing a partner. These games are very good for raising energy and getting people to work with each other. At the end of each go, ask the person on the end of one of the lines to move to the other end so everyone gets a new partner each time.

Yes/No

Duration about 30 seconds to a minute.

One partner's word is *yes*, the other partner's word is *no*; any pair of opposites will create an interesting variation, e.g. *you will – I won't, work – play, indulge – transcend, discipline – freedom, rebel – conform, silly – sensible, think – feel* and so on. Make up your own to suit the circumstances.

This is a good energy raiser and is also good for encouraging shy and quiet people to let out some noise, aided by the more extrovert members of the group. One thing to stress – *no physical contact*. Good-natured folks have been known to get quite wild when entering fully into this game!

Mimicry

Two lines face each other to make pairs, with one line being the speaker and the other the mimic. The leader gives the subject, perhaps a topical one, to the group.

The line of speakers proceeds to talk and gesture, while the mimics imitate them in word and gesture as immediately as possible. It becomes like a mirror image, i.e. no matter what you say and do, you get the same reflected back.

Duration: about 45 seconds to a minute.

Then swap roles – the other line becomes the speakers/ mimics.

A good way to get a spontaneous subject is to ask the team who are to be mimics what they would like their partners to talk about. If someone says 'sex' – and someone usually does – and someone else maybe says 'warthogs' and someone else 'the weather', you can create comical subjects like: 'weather and the sexual habits of warthogs'.

Topical subjects are good too, e.g. 'The joys of Christmas with the family', or at Halloween 'Why I love to bite necks', or at New Year, 'This year's unkeepable resolutions'.

There are many interesting variations, for example:

GIBBERISH
Good for subjects which might be embarrassing in normal language! Or just for the fun of using this profound form of communication.

MOCK OPERA
Sing your 'talk' in mock operatic style.

Car Wash

Get the group into two lines, kneeling, with just enough room between them for a person to crawl down the middle.

One at a time, each person becomes a 'car' and crawls through the car wash and gets 'washed' (gently massaged). Invite them to announce what kind of vehicle they are before coming through.

For example, 'I'm a Jaguar, I'm a pink Mini, I'm a vintage Bentley, I'm a Leyland bus, 97 horse power'.

This is a great game for encouraging touch and helping people to let go of fear of touch. Put on some nice music quietly in the background.

Wild Warm Ups!

Tag Freeze

Someone is 'It'. As in ordinary tag, she chases to touch another, who then becomes 'It'.

The new 'It' freezes, standing with legs apart and arms up.

Anyone else can 'unfreeze' him by crawling through his legs! If the group is large, it works better with several 'Its' at once.

Pat Bottoms

This one comes from Will Schutz and is definitely a touch of California!

Get everyone moving around the space really quickly – get a measure of excitement in the air. Then tell them to look at all the bottoms moving around and as one passes by, to gently pat it!

In a moment or two, with any luck, everyone is running around like crazy patting others on the bottom while trying to avoid being on the receiving end! This game brings the group energy right up. Watch out for anyone going over the top and keep it short.

And an easy one to follow with is:

Stop – Go

Shout 'Stop!' blow your whistle, bang gong, (or whatever you've got) to bring the chaos of the last game to order.

Tell the group that when you say '*Start*', everyone moves, and when you say '*Stop*', everyone stops. (Don't worry if they look at you as if you've gone simple.) Do it a couple of times to get the idea across.

Then tell them this is a game to develop eyes which see behind and to the side, as well as in front, because from now on there are no instructions. As soon as anyone moves, all move. As soon as anyone stops, all stop.

The leader then moves to begin the game. As soon as it is going well, introduce sounds to go with the movement. Later on the sounds can become words.

I like to encourage people to say what they are thinking, and I find that if I do this myself by tuning in to what some of the group are feeling, it triggers others to follow suit, for example 'I could just do with a pint!' or 'This is a very weird kind of game!'

Often, some very funny dialogues ensue, accompanied by a lot of energy being released (and a lot of laughter).

Trust Games
Reed in the Wind

Split into groups of about five to nine people.

One person goes into the centre of each group, and the others make a close circle around her. The one in the middle closes her eyes and relaxes, though keeping straight backed, and lets herself fall gently into the waiting arms of the circle.

The circle supports her and she falls backwards, forwards and sideways like a leaf in the wind.

Duration: about two minutes for each player to go into the centre.

Put on gentle music in the background.

Falling into Someone's Arms

Get everyone to partner up with someone roughly their own size and weight. One stands behind the other so that the partner in front can fall backwards into the waiting arms of the one behind. The front partner raises his arms outward slightly and lets himself fall backwards. The partner behind puts arms out to catch him under his arms as he falls.

This can be quite confronting for some people who have difficulty with trust. Don't be surprised if it brings up some fears. Be aware of safety. Here is a little warning story. When I was living in California in the late 70s, I remember taking part in this game when the leader, who was very much into openness, honesty and being 'in the moment' California-style, told us that it was entirely up to how the catcher felt in that moment as to whether they caught their partner. One person took this literally and let his partner fall onto her back on the hard stone floor. Not a good idea and you need to be sure it doesn't happen.

Falling from a Height (Advanced)

Find a table or some solid place around four to six feet high.

Get about 8 to 12 people together in two lines, facing each other about two feet apart.

Ask them to link arms with the person opposite, with their hands around each other's wrists to make a solid 'bed' between them. They then lean slightly back so as not to be hit on the head.

The participants then, one at a time, take a turn at falling from the table onto the waiting arms! This can be falling forward or backward.

This is a whole degree more advanced. It's good to increase the height slowly as people get used to it, though well within the strength of the catchers. Probably the most challenging for the majority of people is falling backwards with their eyes closed! *Be very aware of safety.*

Blind Lead

In pairs, one partner closes his eyes and the other leads him around, stopping every so often to give him a tactile experience e.g. curtains, radiator, door handle, flowers, chair, fabric etc.

You might choose to put some special unexpected objects around the room, or put some objects in unusual places, or upside down perhaps. Quiet atmospheric music helps.

Also it can be done as an imaginary journey with a voice over: 'You are now walking through a dark forest…crossing a fast flowing river…approaching a dark castle…', etc.

Alternatively, this game can be played outside in nature.

And a nice one to close a trust session is:

Octopus Massage

Get everyone into groups of, say, four to seven.

One person lies down and is massaged by the rest.

Add some gentle music and dim lights. See that everyone has about the same amount of time and ring a bell to indicate changeover.

Ways of Getting into Sub-Groups

Tell everyone to, 'Make groups of five!' then, 'Make groups of three/eight/nine!' etc.

The participants rush about getting into groups of the number you call.

It doesn't matter if anyone is left out. When you have got the groups you desire, end it. This is also a good warm up game in its own right.

Points on the Floor

Ask everyone to get into groups of a chosen size with just a certain number of points touching the floor, e.g. 'Make groups of seven with five points on the floor!'

Everyone gets into groups and attempts to balance so only five points are touching the floor. This usually involves a certain amount of negotiation and hilarity.

Pack of Cards

I call this the Great Spirit's way of forming groups!

Ask everyone to move towards the centre of the room and close their eyes, turn around and then shuffle themselves like a pack of cards. When they are well shuffled, ring the bell to stop and ask them to put out their hands, open their eyes and the first person they connect with is their partner. Sort out the unpaired ones yourself.

four

HELPING PEOPLE
TO MEET

Mingling Games

These are simple role-play exercises to get people in the early shy stages to come together and relate to each other in a fun way. These are 'breaking-down-the-barriers' games.

Cocktail Party – The British Sword and Shield Game

(This game is dated by its inclusion of cigarettes – in its day it was most appropriate!)

This is a joke on us socially-inhibited British as we go out, armed and armoured with our neuroses, to meet others, armed and armoured with theirs, to engage in polite conversation over sherry or cocktails, cigarette firmly in hand.

Ask everyone to put out their right hand as if it held a drink. Tell them this is their shield.

Then ask them to put out their left hand as if it held a cigarette. This is their sword.

Then, armed with the protection of sword and shield, they are at a cocktail party and, being British (or pretending to be) they naturally have just three questions to ask of the others:

'What's your name? Where do you come from? What do you do?'

Then invite them, within those parameters, to meet each other 'intimately' and have 'deep, meaningful conversations'!

This usually encourages a splendid amount of overacting and hilarity.

This can be followed by inviting people to actually meet in twos, threes, or fours for real conversations.

Suspicious

When people first come together, the most frequent inner feelings (likely to be denied by the intellect) are suspicion and fear, and the inner dialogue often goes:

'Will they like me? Do I look OK? Will I be made to look a fool? They all look very confident, unlike me.'

The other side of that can be:

'They all look rather weird. I wonder if there is anyone here I might like? I wonder if I should have stayed home.'

When we are afraid of being rejected, we often tend to reject first. So a good thing is to bring all that out into the open.

Get people to mingle, looking suspiciously at each other.

Stop, meet someone and voice your suspicion.

Move on to someone else and repeat.

Anger Release

After fear there is a natural reaction of anger. One can see this mechanism in animals, but we humans busily cover up our natural instincts and emotions so effectively that most of us have forgotten what they are. These games work when we follow our natural instincts.

Ask everyone to mingle angrily.

And then to find someone to growl at. Then someone else, until they have growled at enough people. Don't go on too long.

VARIATION

1. Grab the next person by the shoulders and shake her a little while growling menacingly. (Be careful that the shaking doesn't become too enthusiastic.)

2. Become a monster and meet another monster. Exchange greetings in monster gibberish.

Culinary Insults

A nice continuation of the last game is insults; not the typical ones, however. The version I like is Culinary Insults (Thanks to Keith Johnstone), i.e. the foulest thing said might be:

A: You filthy rotten egg on mouldy toast!

Countered by:

B: Mouldy toast? You twisted rolling pin.

A: Rolling pin? You foul-mouthed empty jar of rotten carrot juice.

B: Carrot juice? Don't you dare call me carrot juice, you stinking emaciated roll of last year's used kitchen towel!

After playing this in pairs all at once, if the mood is right it makes a great 'competitive' game. Organise the group into teams and play it one pair at a time like a boxing match, with points for the foulest insult and lots of audience encouragement!

Sadness

Invite everyone to act their sadness.

Get some wailing going and encourage overacting.

Find a partner to enjoy a moment of grief with.

This needs to be quite short. You are not attempting to touch deep sadness; this is a role-play.

The Sadness game is a good preparation for the next stage, which is…

Joy

Now ask everyone to meet others with great joy. Tell them that here in the group is the person they most want to meet, the old friend who brings them the most joy. Find someone and act out a joyful meeting.

Compassion

After anger is released, compassion (lovingness) can be expressed. Invite the group to meet each other in a state of compassion.

This is quite difficult and may be better left out at this stage if the group is an inhibited one. Compassion is *not* pity. It is not sentimental, it is not about caring in the do-gooder sense. Compassion is a state of inner stillness from which we can attend to the need of another. This is really an advanced exercise for a 'together' group. There is no 'right way' to do it and it is unteachable in any direct way.

There are myriad ways of bringing people together at the beginning of a session. Here are a few more:

Nationalities

Pretend to be Italian and 'letta your armsa speaka for you. Letta yourself express witha lotta actiona happening and meeta fewa other crazy peoplez'.

Or, think of yourself as Inspector (or Inspectoress) Clouseau and become thoroughly French. Have a deeply French conversation with someone else. (What, you don't speak French? Nor does Inspector Clouseau!)

Similarly, speak in German/Greek/Spanish or any other language. Also, let us not forget that great universal language Glossolalia, otherwise known as gibberish!

This can be played in Cocktail Party format (see first game in this series).

Local Characters

Become a smooth politician/greedy banker/born-again preacher/ East End cockney/Scouser (Liverpudlian)/BBC newsreader/fascist dictator/wimp/pleader/blamer/rationalist/critic/judge/cool/punk/ mafioso/see-the-light evangelist/drugged out rock 'n' roller/ encyclopaedia salesman.

Make your own list to suit local conditions!

Singers

Another great warm up is to do the same in song.

Mock opera/Gregorian chant/country and western/rap/rock n' roll/torch song/jazz.

For example:

A politician singing in mock opera: 'Vote for meeee… I say – you there – you will vote for me, won't you?'

And the partner might respond, 'Vote for you-oo, don't be ridiculous, I will vote for another.'

'Shame upon you-oo. It is I who deserves your vo-ote and your lo-ove.'

Quack

'It's a great ice-breaker, it's never failed me even when working with a cautious group. And you can't get sillier than this!'

TRISHA WOOD

Everyone stands with legs apart, body hanging over forwards and hands on thighs or knees. Then, looking back between the legs, walk around backwards. When you meet someone, exchange the greeting 'Quack!'

Parties

KIDS (7–11 YEARS OLD)

This is suitable for a warmed-up group, and as a free form structure it can be creative and hilarious. It can also bring back very poignant memories of earlier times.

Invite everyone to mingle and lose years until they feel as if they are back in childhood.

Walk and talk like kids at a party. Your body is young, light, sensual – tactile but not sexual. Interact and play with each other like you did when you were children.

Perhaps you play a kids' game with them like Ring-a-Ring-o'-Roses. If you have some chocolate or cakes (and don't mind a mucky floor), this makes a good prop to help them into the feeling of being kids at a party. Keep an eye on the proceedings, while being part of it yourself, as it can get remarkably boisterous. (Don't stand aside or they will relate to you as a parent.)

ADOLESCENTS (14–18 YEARS OLD)

After cleaning up the mess, invite the group to grow up into puberty, to begin to look at the other sex as different, to remember how it was to be a teenager, with a body going through changes, the boys' voices deepening and so on. Put on some rock music…

You are at a teenagers' party. You've all come together to have a great time. The bar is over there (indicate an imaginary bar) and there is music and dancing…

Now just wait and see what a difference this makes! Usually people become shy, inhibited and awkward. Be sure to join in yourself but keep a wary leader's eye on the proceedings.

PARENTS (SEE ALSO COCKTAIL PARTY PREVIOUSLY)

Invite the group to age by about 30 years and to become parents, whatever that means to them. Perhaps they are responsible and mature, or perhaps they have somewhat given up their dreams.

Walk as a parent, find your stance, posture, attitude, the feeling in your body. Feel the responsibility of being a parent. What does it mean to you to relate to others as a parent? Interact and have meaningful contact with other parents. Talk about your children.

If it feels right, put on some old-fashioned dance music, perhaps a waltz. If this is not their 'thing', try some 70s or 80s music or whatever period the group will relate to as 'parental'.

OURSELVES

We are at our own party, here and now, as ourselves. (Think that's easy? Try it!)

ALTERNATIVE

It is an interesting alternative to play this sequence backwards, i.e. start with parents, regress to teenagers, then kids and finally back to ourselves.

There is a lot to be learned from this seemingly simple sequence. Open sharing around the circle can be very advantageous at the end.

five
VERBAL IMPROVISATION GAMES

These are games to develop spontaneity and creativity and to let the imagination flow unfettered. They are vehicles for self-development which can contribute greatly to freedom from the censor inside us. In our culture we are very good at empowering the critic. Many of us have been so criticised that we do not dare to speak before thinking, and so we kill our own spontaneity and creativity. Then when we perform, we judge our performance harshly, so it can take time, effort and persistence to improvise really well. However, there is a 'secret'.

The Secret of Improvisation

I often ask people at a workshop to put up their hands if they feel they are experts at improvisation, and usually only a few do, if any. I then ask those who think they are not experts and have little or no experience to put up their hands, and usually lots of hands go up. I then get quite serious and ask who handed them their 'life script' when they plopped into this world out of the womb, and have they been following it ever since? And, furthermore, are they working to their script right now?

'What! You mean you're making your life up as you go along? You're improvising!' The penny drops amid laughter, and I make the point that we are all experts at improvisation because we do it all the time.

All our lives are an improv!

Theatre improvisation is merely a change of setting for something we are all naturally expert at. I have seen great changes in people who thought they couldn't improvise, once this point got home.

Word Games
Story Round

This is the old kids' game. I use these variations:

Someone starts a story and hands it on when ready.

The next person adds as much as he feels like and then hands it on, and so on.

Or, each person adds up to six words.

Or, each person says only one word.

With the last variation it is quite difficult to get a story which makes sense, so I find it works better to start with the first two versions. Sometimes I have found this game really hilarious and at other times sticky. I tend to use it with a warmed-up group.

Fortunately/Unfortunately

One person begins a sentence with, 'Fortunately, so and so…'

The next butts in, 'But unfortunately,…' and adds to the first person's statement.

The following person says, 'But fortunately,…' and recounts something which puts the situation to rights.

For example:

Jack: Fortunately, I ate a good meal tonight.

Liz: But unfortunately, it was heavily laced with poison, and I'm dying.

Tara: But fortunately, there was a doctor in the house with a handy stomach pump.

Bill: But unfortunately, he was an animal doctor, and the pump was for an elephant.

And so on…

This game can be played in pairs or in a circle.

It is important to add to the action each time and not to repeat a situation.

The elements here are speed, non-censoring of the imagination, lateral thinking and illogical logic. There is no need whatsoever to make sense; the keynote is permission to express. Whatever anyone says is right, and the group will learn through this and similar games provided that they are always supported by the leader and never criticised.

Yes, But

This is really a variation of the last game. One person makes a statement and the next butts in, 'Yes, but…' and so on.

For example:

Abdul: I have been feeling quite healthy these past few days.

Chris: Yes, but my corns hurt when I put my feet on the ground.

Joel: Yes, but with these ropes to hold me up, I don't have to touch the ground.

Chan: Yes, but they keep breaking because I'm 24 stone.

Babs: Yes, but with my new slimming regime I'll be so light soon it won't matter.

No, You Didn't!

1. AS A GAME IN PAIRS

Partner 'A' tells a story of something that happened. For example: 'This is what I did yesterday.'

After a sentence or two, partner 'B' butts in: 'No, you didn't!'

Partner 'A' apologises for lying and tells a different story: 'I'm sorry, you're quite right. This is what really happened…'

It develops rather like a person telling fibs, getting into hot water and then making more and more elaborate excuses to try to get out of the mess.

2. AS A CIRCLE GAME

The story remains in the first person as it goes around the circle no matter who is telling it, so one person tells a story, then the next chooses a moment to butt in and says, 'No you didn't.'

The following person in the circle apologises and carries on with a new story.

Never Mind That, Tell Me About…

This is similar to the previous games and can be played in partners or in a circle. First let's look at it as a circle game.

The first person talks about something.

The next butts in, 'Never mind that, tell me about…', picking up the subject from the first person's monologue.

The third person then takes over, and so on.

This game needs an uneven number so that everyone has a chance to be the 'teller'. If there is an even number in the group, the leader takes either both roles or neither when her turn comes, so that participants get alternating roles.

Alternatively like the others mentioned previously, it can be played very successfully as a partner game.

For example:

'Did you know that UFOs colonised the earth millennia ago and we are really a genetic experiment?'

'Never mind that, tell me about genetic.'

'Genetic is when things are passed down and…'

'Never mind that, tell me about passed down.'

'Passed down is what happened to me when I was just a little boy and I was passed down and out and there was no hope for poor me.'

'Never mind that, tell me about hope.'

The Meaning of Life

A standing circle. Someone moves into the centre and gives his opinion of the meaning of life. (Inevitably it's often '42'!)

After a sentence or two, someone picks up on something he has said and takes the first person's place. He then states his view. (The first person yields and rejoins the circle.)

Here's an example:

First person: The meaning of life is graciousness and good manners and tea. The true meaning of life can always be found over a nice cuppa.

Second person: Rubbish, the meaning of life is money, money, money and owning everything.

Third person: Don't be so materialistic, the meaning of life is clean air, it's all in the breath.

Fourth person: Clean air? We haven't got any clean air and we're still alive so don't talk rubbish. The meaning of life is chocolate. Without chocolate we'd all die in agony.

This is a very simple format and the game can be hilarious provided rational logic doesn't get a hold! With the Play-World group it tends to resemble the *Hitchhiker's Guide to the Galaxy*. The art of this game is in picking up on something said and taking it to another extreme of absurdity.

Good News and Bad News

A similar format to The Meaning of Life. One person comes into the circle and tells some 'good' news. Anyone else comes in and interrupts with some relevant 'bad' news, while the first person rejoins the circle. Then someone else comes in with good news and so on.

For example:

'The good news is that it's lovely and warm today.'

'But the bad news is the whole planet is warming and it will be too hot to live here soon.'

'Ah, but the good news is that England will soon be sub-tropical.'

'And the bad news is there is going to be a pole shift and sub-tropical regions will be under snow at the poles!'

You're Lucky! (Based on the Monty Python Sketch)

Again a similar format.

One person goes into the middle and complains bitterly about something!

Another participant in the circle, picks up on something said, and exclaims, 'You're lucky', enters the circle and takes over with a diatribe about how much more terrible his life is, and so it goes on.

Like this…

'I have to work 20 hours a day digging the road just to earn a crust of bread.'

'You're lucky to have a job, mate, I have to beg all day and night just to get a cuppa tea.'

'You can beg? You're so lucky! I never had the opportunity to be real like that. My family is so rich it's stultifying. There are so many appearances to keep up that it's like being in prison.'

'You're rich? You're lucky to be rich. I'd go to prison for a decent meal.'

'A decent meal! Sheer luxury. I live on scraps from the gutter. A decent meal for me is a good worm flavoured with bird droppings.'

We also play this as a theatre improv 'on stage'. It is a good way of promoting non-logical thought and can be a vehicle for a group to take off into wild and splendid fantasy.

Creative Excuses

The leader blames one member of the circle for something (avoiding personal issues). This person then makes creative excuses for having done whatever it is, and then blames the next person in such a way that he becomes the 'real' culprit, and so on around the circle while the excuses get more and more complicated and bizarre.

The fun in this game comes from keeping a thin thread of logic and stretching it.

Painting an Elephant

This is a game of lateral thinking.

One person mimes a common movement in the centre of the circle. The next person asks, 'What are you doing?' The first replies anything except what he is actually doing.

For example:

The first person mimes cleaning windows.

'What are you doing?' asks the second.

'Painting an elephant!' replies the first.

The second person then mimes painting an elephant.

The next person asks, 'What are you doing?'

The second person replies, 'Checking the traffic lights to see if they are green.'

The third person then mimes checking traffic lights – and so on around the circle.

Murder! or Killer Wink!

The group is in a standing circle facing inwards. The leader asks everyone to close their eyes and then walks around the outside of the circle and touches one person secretly on the back. This person is the murderer.

The group then mingle, pretending perhaps to be at an Agatha Christie-style house party. The murderer's weapon is a devastating '*wink!*' and he endeavours to 'murder' someone so that no one else sees who is doing the dastardly deed.

The murdered person counts to four before dying in some wonderfully dramatic way. The group continue to mingle, and murders continue, until someone thinks he's sussed out the murderer, when he says 'I accuse…' and names who he thinks it is. The leader lets him know if he is right or wrong. The game continues until the murderer is unmasked.

Last – two facility training games.

Word Challenge

Yes this is a challenging game! The rule is you can say any word except the one just spoken. Seems simple? Try it and see!

Make a standing circle of 6–12 people. If the group is larger, make two circles.

The leader begins by saying *any* word and points to someone in the circle.

That person then says *any other word* and points to someone else, and so on.

Easy? At slow speed, yes. But this is a fast game, and the idea is to get faster and faster, firing words at one another. This is a game of skill-development and of freeing the mind, stopping the censor within. It is not just a fun game but one which develops mental freedom and spontaneity. Try it and see how fast you can go before you trip yourself up.

Back to Front (thanks to Ian Kalman)

Get the group walking around the space, aware of each other.

Tell them to *stop* – and they *stop*. Tell them to *go* – and they *go*…

Then instruct them that when you say 'stop', they *go*, and when you say 'go', they *stop*!

Try this out till they've got it – the command means its opposite.

Next, tell them to *jump up in the air* – and they do so – and tell them to *clap hands* – and they do that too. Then instruct them to do the reverse of that too! *Jump up* means clap hands and vice-versa.

You now have four commands and you have organised the group to respond oppositely to each of them.

Play with it – start slowly and speed up – it is much harder to do than it seems and gets interesting results as it challenges our automatic responses.

six
THEATRE GAMES AND IMPROVISATIONS

TV Off, Creativity On!

In our society we have largely replaced homemade entertainment with TV, movies, professional theatre, professional concerts and so on. We have tended largely to give our power away to 'experts' as if only other people can entertain adequately. Today, there is rarely home entertainment in the way that there used to be. Play-World is about bringing back that tradition and we have had some of the most stomach-aching belly laughing sessions of theatre games, and times when the most unlikely people have found previously hidden abilities and talents.

What follows are games and structures which work well when played 'on stage'.

Invite the group to sit down as the 'audience', leaving a suitable space in front for people to come up and perform. Tell them the gist of what you are going to do and, if necessary, talk a little about improvisation and how natural it is. (See 'The Secret of Improvisation' at the beginning of Chapter 5.)

Machines

This is a well-known game, a good energy mover and good for beginning theatre improv.

One person comes out front and makes a mechanical sound and movement.

Another joins in with an appropriate additional sound and movement.

Others join, one at a time, until the machine is made.

Five to eight people is a good number for this, even ten at a pinch.

VARIATIONS

1. 'Freeze' the action and ask the audience to suggest an emotion for the machine. The machine then 'gets emotional'.

2. Freeze the action and ask the audience for the function of this machine – the more ridiculous the better – e.g. 'It's a machine for mending invisible holes in the road' or 'It's for assembling giraffes' heads to their bodies'.

The machine attempts to carry out its purpose.

'A tap with a hammer, a turn with a spanner… All machines can go wrong and now from working perfectly, the machine breaks down…'

After about a half to one minute, as soon as the energy peaks, ring the bell for the end.

Cartoons and Captions

About three to seven members come out front and make a still picture like a cartoon. The audience suggest captions.

Movie Stills

About three to seven members come out front, and this time they make a still scene from a movie. The audience guess what it is.

Then the players come to life and create a short scene (a half to one minute).

Statuary

Again, about three to seven people come out front.

The audience suggest who the players are, e.g. footballers/politicians/great lovers/punks/bankers/pop group/layabouts/accountants/fascists/preachers/lager louts. The players then silently make a still picture of whatever they are given.

On a ring of the bell the picture comes to life and they create a short scene (about a half to one-and-a-half minutes usually seems about right).

VARIATIONS

1. Add an emotion, e.g. happy undertakers/loving fascists/miserable lovers.

2. The leader asks two questions of the audience: 'Who are they?' and 'What are they doing right now?' For example, they are a pop group trying to write a hit song/prison warders discussing how to help a troublesome prisoner to escape/preachers discussing which one is most holy.

Paranoid

This one came to me spontaneously one night and worked brilliantly. The title is quite illogical but that is what we called it then and so that's what it's been called ever since! It is a great game to get things moving.

There are about four to eight players on stage.

Invite the audience to give them an emotion. They then have 30–40 seconds to play that emotion to the *fullest*!

Leave the rules as loose as possible. Can they relate to each other or to the rest of the group (the audience), as well? Yes! Encourage them to let rip and *overact* all the way…and as soon as the energy crescendoes, ring the bell for the end.

Interruptions (Requirements: Two Chairs)

Put two chairs side by side. Invite four people up, two to sit on the chairs and two to stand behind them.

Ask the audience for a controversial topic for discussion.

The two sitting then discuss the topic. One is for and the other against.

The two behind are the directors and when they tap the speaker in front of them on the shoulder he changes view instantly and argues the opposite position.

This is hilarious when the two speakers really get into it – the sudden changes of opinion, and the effort involved in trying to make the changes sound reasonable, create a lot of fun. They can sound horribly like real politicians doing U-turns and denying they have done so! It also can remind us how many TV and radio debates are set up as controversies between people arguing from set positions where there can be no coming together or real meeting, just a fudging of the issues.

Keystone Cops (Requirements: Four or Five Chairs)

Most people know the zany exploits of the Keystone Cops and their wonderfully hopeless inefficiency.

Get four chairs and five people on stage (or five chairs and six people).

The Keystone Cops are hanging around when, on the sound of the whistle, they see a baddie on the run and rush to their 'car' (the chairs) and set off in pursuit – with everything in sight going wrong, of course.

You need a good one-minute piece of 1920s honky-tonk music. (I use 'Grandma's Spells', the Jelly Roll Morton piano piece from the 1920s.)

This game is a boisterous romp in knockabout comedy mode and can release lots of energy and laughter. There's not much 'point' to it; it simply helps people get into 'the ridiculous'.

Interviews (Requirements: Two Chairs)

Two people sit out front. One is the interviewer and the other the interviewee.

Ask the audience for a topic and a style for the interviewer. The style can be that of any well-known person.

You can ask the audience for questions or leave it to the interviewer.

VARIATIONS

1. Mr Expert: The interviewee is an expert and thus knows all the answers – however unlikely they may be.

2. Three-Headed Expert: Three people are one expert. Each says only one word at a time and answers in rotation the

question put by the interviewer. Or, the three have to speak all at once, saying the same words!

One Minute Please – Simple Version

This one is a well-known game.

One person comes out front and asks for a topic and then speaks on it for a minute.

One Minute Please – Slightly More Advanced Version

As in the simple version previously, but without hesitation, repetition or deviation.

One-Minute Commercial

It's nice to have a collection of unlikely items for this one!

One person comes on stage and is given an item and a minute to 'sell' it.

Alternatively, if you do not have objects, the audience can suggest imaginary items.

Unusual Sporting Events

Ask the audience for an everyday activity, e.g. doing the washing up.

Ask for four people to come up.

Two people mime the activity while the other two give an animated commentary, sports-style.

Foreign Movies (Requirements: Two Chairs)

Invite four people up.

Two create a scene using the wonderful language of gibberish, pausing between lines so that the other two can give subtitles to the movie!

Hidden Agendas (Also Requires Two Chairs)

This is a similar idea to Foreign Movies.

Using four people, the two centre stage create a scene with words, which are preferably highly emotional. The other two, from the side, supply the hidden thoughts!

Highly-charged romance, with a touch of Ingmar Bergman, works really well for this.

Freeze (Requirements: Two Chairs or Settee or Similar)

This is a great little structure for two players. It probably comes from Viola Spolin who was the originator of much of this kind of work. Her book, *Improvisation for the Theater* (1999), is still a classic.

Two players on stage create a scene.

Anyone else in the group can shout 'Freeze!' at any time.

The players freeze in whatever physical position they are in, and the new player replaces either one, taking up the same physical position but starting a new scene. And so it continues.

This structure is so simple, yet much can be done with it and much can be learned from it. One of the issues that comes up is that of people getting anxious about when to say 'freeze' and what might happen if they get up on stage and don't know what to do. This brings to the surface the old problems of 'Am I doing it right?', 'Am I good enough?', 'Everyone else will do it OK except me', etc., and I like to work with this in several ways. First, to specifically encourage people not to think before saying 'freeze', and to remember that if they do find themselves 'on stage' and don't know what to say, they can say what is true at that moment, 'I don't know what to say', or, 'I don't know what I'm doing here'. Both of these are great opening lines and give the partner lots of options as to how to respond.

The second way is for the group to 'freeze' each other, i.e. say 'freeze' and indicate another member of the group who goes on stage.

In this way no one knows when they will find themselves up there.

At one workshop where we were working specifically with fears, these were a few of the responses to being 'freezed' by someone else. Peter said, 'I found it easier. I found it better because I didn't have a preconceived idea.' John said, 'I felt under less pressure because I could blame the person who sent me up!' Paul said, 'I find it much easier if somebody drops me in it.'

It really is amazing how we frustrate our own creative process with anxiety. Most of us who teach this kind of work, and therapeutic work in general, are teaching things we need to learn. The more I teach, the clearer things become to me. I consider myself a student in my own classes and workshops, and this helps me to keep my feet on the ground and my head out of the clouds!

There are many variations to try, for example:

NAMES FREEZE

The players open by addressing each other with a name, preferably evocative of something; 'Good morning, Mr Snide', 'Good morning, Mrs Mothering'. A sketch proceeds, with the players taking their character from the name they are given.

Then 'freeze', and a new player replaces one of the protagonists.

'Hello, is your name Eric Beanworthy?'

'Yes, and I see from your name tag that you are Mr Disappointed.'

'Yes, I'm afraid so. Nothing ever seems to go right for me.'

And so on.

At the end of each sketch, both characters can be dropped and new ones taken up.

THERAPIST – CLIENT FREEZE

Each sketch involves therapist and client, but there is no rule as to which is to be which. That is allowed to emerge in the dialogue, and it is sometimes surprising how it does, and who is which.

Alternatively, one chair is the therapist's and the other the client's.

LOVERS' FREEZE

Each scene involves two lovers.

OPERA-LOVERS FREEZE

The whole sketch takes place in mock opera-style. Never mind if anyone 'can sing' – that has nothing to do with it!

Let it rip – in tune, out of tune, sung or spoken. Nothing matters except that it is hilariously overacted.

Make up your own variation of it: politicians/mock blood and thunder evangelists/parents/children/villains.

NEWSPAPER FREEZE

Have a newspaper handy and give it to the players. The first line of every sketch is to be any line from the newspaper which one player reads out spontaneously. What they do with it after that is up to them.

For example:

Player A: *(Reads.)* Britons were targeted and lured away by Texas sect. *(This refers to the Waco siege in Texas, 28 February – 19 April 1993.)*

Player B: They tried to get me when I went into the Texas store up the road, but I insisted I just wanted to buy some curtain rail.

Player A: You were lucky to get out. I was terrified when I went into B&Q and I only wanted some nails. Mind you, Sainsbury's is the worst. Have you been to their garden centre? They tried to get right inside my head with a lawn mower!

Or:

Player A: *(Reads a headline.)* Academics tackle computer babel.

Player B: I know. It's not been the same since the invention of talking computers. They won't shut up, you know. Mine keeps telling me off – it's worse than having a wife. And it doesn't even do the washing up!

This is a good structure to relieve anxiety in a shy group, because it gets rid of the first line 'What should I say?' worries. It can also be very funny, as it can bring topical issues into the action.

SHAKESPEAREAN FREEZE

All action is spoken and acted in mock Shakespeare-style. As an example, this excerpt is from the Play-World show *The Great Improvisation*, November 1985.

Francesca: Sire, look ye yonder. *(Pointing towards audience.)*

Joe: Verily, many faces have come to see thy figure…and my heart. *(Preens himself.)*

Francesca: No, sire, this is your heart. *(Puts her hand on his heart.)*

Joe: It may be my heart, madam, but t'was not in my thoughts…my thoughts stream down my body like a plague when I see thee. May I speak plain to thee?

Francesca: Nay, sire.

Joe: So plain that it be disgusting, madam.

Francesca: Nay, nay, sire.

Joe: Give me your hand…and let me have the rest of you by tonight. Say aye, say aye, say aye.

Francesca: Nay.

Joe: Then I go to kill myself. I bring forth this dagger…

Francesca: Nay, take… *(She mumbles and cannot be heard for audience laughter.)*

Joe: Take thy what, madam? Speak thy words fluently, or get off!

Freeze.

Robert comes on and takes Francesca's place.

Robert: *(Taking on an upper-class, high-status character.)* Who are you and what are you doing, my man?

Joe: *(Adopting underdog character suggested by Robert's opening line.)* I've come from the fields a muck spreading, as a muck spreading I shall surely go, sire.

Robert: Did you see Cornwall's army advancing as you spread your muck?

Joe: Only Daisy the cow, sire.

Like all the previous improv games, this is a spontaneous happening. Obviously it is only suitable for a group of people with some knowledge of Shakespearean style and content.

Merry-Go-Round

This is a similar two-hander to Freeze, but instead of freezing and starting a new sketch, the new player joins in the existing action, and one of the current players finds a way to exit.

Two players on stage create a sketch. At any time an additional player can join in. Then one of the first two players finds a way, within the action of the sketch, to make an exit.

VARIATION

Have more players on stage. For example, set the basic number at three with a fourth entering and one or two of the three finding a way to exit.

This is also a very nice, easy structure to work with. I find some groups thrive more on Freeze, and others on this one. An alternative is to play it in the centre of a standing circle.

Lovers

This was previously mentioned as a way to play Freeze but it is also good to play as separate sketches. The main difference is that the leader must signal the end when she feels the game has run its course.

I have sometimes created a bedroom set with mattresses and pillows for this game. The results have been both poignant and humorous, and a great many insights have occurred to the participants. We always spend time sharing feelings afterwards with very healing results.

Dying a Death

This is a great game for encouraging people to really let go. Definitely one from OA. That's 'Overactors Anonymous'!

There are two players. One starts by saying something quite insipid. But it is so devastating to the other that he goes into a magnificent death scene. With the last breath the 'dying' player utters a word (any word) which is so devastating to the first player that he is unable to do anything but 'die' hysterically too!

End of scene. Next two players, please!

Body Language (Before Words)

Two players are on stage, preferably seated. Each player expresses herself physically before uttering a word.

For example:

Man and woman sitting next to each other.

Woman looks surreptitiously at man.

He turns to look at her.

She looks away quickly, pretending disinterest.

He looks into the distance.

She slowly turns towards him.

Then he turns towards her.

They find themselves eye to eye.

'Er…', he says shyly.

She turns away quickly. 'I was wondering…,' he says.

No reply.

He turns away and pretends to be preoccupied.

She looks at him, inspecting him.

Pause.

He looks at his watch.

'Do you have the time?' she asks.

'Er…no,' he says.

She looks at his watch and then at him. 'You never do, do you?'

He says, 'I was thinking…'

She looks away and crosses her legs away from him.

'Since when have you ever "thought" about anything?' she says.

He turns away quickly and huffily, and crosses his legs.

'It wasn't my fault, really.'

The scene acquires something of a Pinteresque quality and gradually unfolds, with the hidden agendas slowly revealing themselves. It is important that neither player has a 'script' and that the action unfolds bit by bit, and is as much a surprise to them as to the audience. It is amazing just how much can be expressed in this way and how much self-recognition takes place. It can become hilarious when the characters express one thing with their actions and another with their words.

Lecturer and Slides

Three to five players are on stage. Elicit a suitably crazy subject from the audience. One player gives a lecture.

Two (or three or four) players are demonstrators and act out the visuals.

This can also be done with the lecturer describing a picture which the demonstrators then make visual.

The lecturer then says, 'Next slide, please', and the demonstrators create a picture for which he creates a suitably comic description.

For example:

Subject – mountain-climbing under the ocean.

Lecturer begins: I remember the day I undertook the tremendous challenge of climbing the highest mountain under the sea. My friend and I loaded our equipment. Here is a picture of us in the act.

Demonstrators create a visual picture.

Lecturer: Next slide please.

Demonstrators make a new visual.

Ah, and here we are setting off down to the bottom of the ocean.

And so on.

This really comes into the category of a warm up. It is one of the less demanding games, particularly for the demonstrators. The fun is in the interaction between the lecturer and the visuals.

Committees – thanks to Bill Downey
(Requirements: Four to Six Chairs)

When we British want, or more likely don't want, to achieve something, the first thing we do is form a committee. A committee has meetings, and meetings beget meetings, until in the end the main part of the agenda is setting the date for the next meeting. To quote the wonderful Sir Humphrey from the TV series, *Yes, Minister*, 'If you really want to put the whole business on ice, Minister, then form an action committee.'

Invite four to six people out front and then elicit from the audience the name and function of a committee, e.g. a committee for the propagation of meetings.

Ask the players to choose a chairperson.

First, the committee are having their picture taken for the in-house journal. The players pose suitably, all smiles.

Next, let's see the *real* relationships between the committee members. The players pose again. Factions immediately form.

Next, for about a minute or more, let's see the committee in action as the chair person initiates the issue to be discussed.

Ring the bell for the end when it's gone as far as feels right.

Couples

Invite two people on stage. Ask the audience for a relationship between them and an issue that has come up for them.

They create a scene. As soon as the energy reaches a climax or a low, ring the bell for the end.

Therapist and Client

One person is the therapist and the other is the client.

Ask the audience for a well-known figure who is *not* in the therapy world. The therapist then takes on the style of that figure.

I remember some hilarious Play-World scenes of diverse types of therapy in the styles of Basil Fawlty, Hitler, Mrs Thatcher (the client didn't get a look in that time!), Larry Grayson ('Ooo shut that door…!'), David Frost ('Hello, good evening and welcome to your neurosis'), Hercule Poirot and James Bond.

Updated personalities could be Obama, Putin, Joffrey (from *Game of Thrones*), Captain Jack Sparrow (*Pirates of the Caribbean*), etc. It's best to choose famous and distinct personalities of your time and place, and the less they relate to therapy, the better.

Trios

Invite three people up and ask the audience for a relationship and an issue. Or just ask for a situation. They create a spontaneous scene.

A good variation for trios is family scenes.

Ask for three family roles, one for each player, and an issue that has come up. Ring the bell to start the scene.

Character Couples

Make up some cards with the names of comic stereotypical couples. For example:

Valerie and Vic Victim/Bessie and Bert Blamer/Deirdre and Danny Dreamer/Peter and Penny Plan/Pansie and Patrick Poser/ Gloria and George Jealous/Inga and Ian Indulgence/Matthew and Madonna Mystic/Penelope and Paul Perfect/Ryan and Rena Righteous/Tara and Timothy Tragedy/Walter and Winnie Wimp/ Roger and Rita Rescue/Horace and Hetty Holy/Prunella and Percival Prude/Tom and Tina Tyrant.

I am sure you get the idea. Invite four people to come up and divide them into the two couples. Put the cards face down and ask each couple to take one.

Ask the audience for a place and a situation, e.g. neighbours talking over the garden wall, and an issue between them. Let the scene begin.

An alternative scenario is to mix the cards and get the four players to take one each and become the appropriate gender of the card they chose, e.g. Vic Victim might be coupled with Rita Rescue. Very interesting mixes come out of this with lots of room to create comical dramas!

seven

POWER AND
STATUS GAMES

An important area I have not yet mentioned is status games. Keith Johnstone's chapter on this in his book *Impro* (1979) is profound and I refer you to this altogether wonderful book (see Resources). He talks about how we are 'forbidden' to see status transactions except when there is a conflict. For example, in a park we may notice the ducks squabbling, but we probably do not see how carefully they keep their distance when they are not. When we talk about the struggle for status, we are really talking about dominance and submission, even sado-masochism. But to use such terms is to run the risk of being seriously misunderstood.

So let us simply call them status transactions.

We are all hierarchical animals, a fact we rarely acknowledge unless we are on top!

> 'Normal' people are inhibited from seeing that no action, sound or movement is innocent of purpose. Many psychiatrists have noted how uncannily perceptive some schizophrenics are. I think that their madness must have opened their eyes to things that 'normal' people are trained to ignore.
>
> (Johnstone 2012, p.41)

We are all familiar with such classic stereotypes as the henpecked husband and the dominant wife or the high-status husband and 'the little woman', as well as the prolific status transactions of the office, and the rabid laughter which occurs when the boss makes the most pathetic of jokes. Worse still is the office party, so well shown in the wonderful sit-com *The Office*. If we play out these games without awareness it is at our peril. How much better to become aware.

We can observe status players in any walk of life. Here are two from my schooldays, both teachers. One, whom we called 'Botty', was a war veteran who had suffered some injury and only knew how to play low status. He was hopeless at imposing any semblance of discipline and was very nice to us. As a reward the class taunted him horribly. One day he got so angry he hit a boy, rather deservedly, on the head, not very hard. We all shouted, 'Cry, cry!' to the boy, who made a great act of crying. Somehow or other we then proceeded to get this poor old man to apologise to the boy. I hate to look back and think I had anything to do with such a shameful episode. The other teacher we called 'Hoot'; he was an imperiously high-status player and kept fearsome discipline. He taught Latin, and at the time I was in the O Level failures class, due to retake the subject in the autumn. He took a dislike to me – or so it seemed – and sat me in the front of the class right under his beady eye, and then proceeded to ignore me as if I wasn't worth teaching. This ploy obviously worked well because at the end of term exam I passed. The following term the failures again collected in his class and later one of them gleefully told me that Hoot had looked around and asked, 'Where's Rutherford?'

Someone gingerly put up his hand (playing low status with such a teacher is very wise) and said 'I think he passed, sir.' (He knew perfectly well.) 'He's what?' responded Hoot imperiously. I was told the expression on his face was a joy to behold!

Other typical high-status players are military commanders. Some successful commanders have been more terrifying to their troops than the enemy! Leading actors and actresses usually play high status, while 'character actor' is a euphemism for someone who knows how to play low status. I have listed at the end of this chapter the attributes needed to maintain power as suggested by Desmond Morris, author of *The Naked Ape* (1967) and *The Human Zoo* (1969).

The problem for us is to learn to become fully conscious of status games and to know which role someone is playing, to learn to read their motives clearly and to be able, at will, to play whatever status we choose. To become more in command of our own life and less a victim of circumstances and of other people is the essence of personal growth. The majority play status unconsciously – after all, the whole British class system is about status and we are taught to accept it blindly, as if some are superior by divine right. Consider the low-status-playing teacher, like Botty, who does not understand that what he does negates his efforts to maintain discipline, the browbeaten wife who assumes her husband's superiority, and the underdog employee who grovels out of habit. How wonderful to be able to grovel consciously (and be able to laugh inwardly at the situation), but how awful to be brainwashed to believe that this is all you are entitled to do! Everyone who plays victim – low status – attracts to them persecutors – high status. Only when we learn to change ourselves inside do our experiences change in the outer world.

Tragedy and Comedy

'Tragedy is the ousting of the high-status animal from the top of the pack' (Johnstone 2012, p.41).Tragedy is obviously related to sacrifice. Two things strike me about reports of sacrifices: one is that the crowd gets more and more tense, and then relaxes after the moment of death; the other is that the victim is raised in status before being sacrificed. The best goat is chosen and it is groomed and magnificently decorated. A human sacrifice, in stories from long ago, might be pampered for months and then dressed in the finest clothes and rehearsed in his/her role at the centre of the great ceremony. Elements of this can be seen in the Christ story (the robe, the crown of thorns and even the eating of the 'body' in church services). 'A sacrifice has to be endowed with high status or the magic doesn't work' (Johnstone 1979). Shakespeare understood all of this very well, and his tragedies are all about pecking orders and the incredible machinations people go to in order to gain power and status. Today, TV's *Game of Thrones* says it all!

Comedy, too, involves status transactions, and much of it is about pontification and the attempt to gain status, and about what happens when we are found out. Jokes involve either gaining or losing status. To be made a fool of is to lose status; to 'put one over on' someone is to gain status at their expense. Yet when we watch comedy it is only funny when we have sympathy with the underdog. Charlie

Chaplin and Norman Wisdom personify the little man who wins against all odds and beats the high-status players of the world, just as we would like to. French and Saunders are so enjoyable because they are constantly creating a tension of status between them. Consider Morecambe and Wise and the constant putting down of 'Little Ern' by Eric, Ernie constantly having ideas above his station with his ridiculous plays, and how funny it is when he manages to put one over on Eric. Look at the incredible antics of Laurel and Hardy and the battles between them. Status games are central to all successful comedy double acts.

In my experience of workshops, the whole concept of status transactions brings up considerable resistance in people. We are taught not to see them; moreover, our egos won't let us see them because they make us uncomfortable about the extent to which we are not in control and the degree to which we manipulate in order to get through daily life. Nevertheless, we are always the leader or follower in any human interaction and there is no position in between. I have put this across in workshops and encountered enormous resistance. The Dolphin Dance (see Chapter 8) is a simple structure of leader and followers. It simply doesn't work without a leader; it ends in confusion. In the dance everyone gets their moment of being leader (king) and the rest of the time submits to following (courtier), and that can make a beautiful cohesive experience. In this life, if we want to create order, to do something together, some are required to be leaders and many to be followers. When people have disagreed with me about this I have demonstrated it through simple everyday role-play exercises, such as a boy asking a girl out to the cinema. How can one do this without any status being transacted?

Boy: Would you like to come to the movies? (*Can be played with any status.*)

Girl: Which one? (*High status. She wants to have a choice.*)

Boy: Well – er – whichever one you'd like. (*Lowers himself to ensure date.*)

Or:

Boy: I'm going to see *Guns and Butter*. You can come if you like. (*High status – keeping control.*)

Girl: No thanks. (*High status – not going to submit to that!*)

Or:

Boy tries it another way: I'd like to see *Guns and Butter*. It's supposed to be very good. (*Lowers status slightly to encourage her.*)

Girl: I'd quite like to see it, but what about *Drunks in Heaven*? That had a terrific write-up. (*Challenges his status.*)

Boy: You mean the one in *Time Out*? Their reviewers are crazy. A friend saw it and said it was rubbish. (*Upstages her a lot.*)

Girl: Oh alright then, *Guns and Butter*. (*Lowers status. Submits to his will.*)

Or:

> **Girl**: *Drunks in Heaven* is an art film – lots of people don't have what it takes to understand art films. That's what I want to see anyway. (*High status – rubbishes his friend and goes for dominance.*)

If you don't believe me, try out a role-play like this with a friend and see if you can really do it without status transactions. Just the fact of someone's preference being agreed over the other's is enough! In Keith Johnstone's words: 'My answer is that acquaintances become friends when they agree to play status games together' (Johnstone 2012, p.37). (Obviously he means agree sub-consciously.)

How many times have you seen someone get up to talk to an audience and begin by apologising? Or perhaps someone at a party is asked to talk about something they know about and begins, 'Of course I don't really know much, but if you really want me to tell you then…' (Usually the body language gives away just how much they relish the spotlight.) In the year-long course I ran for 20 years, participants got the opportunity early on to sit in front of the group and tell their life story. Always some of them started by apologising for themselves. I call this phenomenon 'insurance'; it is an attempt to insure the future by making excuses for oneself first. It is playing low status in an attempt to ensure that no matter how good you are no one will be jealous, or no matter how bad you are no one will let you know what they really think!

When playing high or low status, there are body movements that speak louder than words. This list comes primarily from Keith Johnstone (2012) but I have added one or two extras.

High status:

- walk tall

- smooth movements

- take a lot of space

- head kept still, especially when talking

- hands kept away from face

- dominant in speech

- sit back and spread yourself

- feel splayed out

- head held high

- inner dialogue: 'Be wary of me, I bite.'

Low status:

- walk small

- jerky movements

- occupy little space

- head moves a lot

- hands go near face a lot

- hesitant – 'ers' and 'ums' in speech

- sit hunched

- toes point inwards

- head bowed

- inner dialogue: 'Please don't bite me, I'm not worth the trouble.'

Talking of status and space, I remember one person I used to know socially, and every time I met him, I would find myself walking slowly backwards as we talked. He invaded my space – and I remember he had bad breath too! We humans have a natural boundary and when people come too close or stay too far away, it doesn't feel right. We are energy bodies, luminous eggs in the words of Castaneda's Don Juan, and we don't like our egg to be invaded unless we choose. Interestingly, the acceptable boundaries of personal space vary from culture to culture.

In this transaction I was playing low status. To change, I would have had to confront him but I didn't want the effort and comeback so I let him get away with it – with the simple intention of staying away from him. That was a long time ago and I might act differently now.

Trisha Wood was running a series of Play-World evenings and it became clear after a bit that whatever role Pete was playing, he took on high status. When he was an underdog, he was a rebel underdog, when playing a worker he always tried to dominate the boss. In the game of Pecking Order (see Status Games) he was quite unable to play No 4. In fact, it didn't matter where he was in the line, he could only play high status. Now at the same time in his personal life, he was unable to keep a job, and had had numerous very short periods of employment. Trish spent a lot of time working with him till he realised what he was doing and learned how to play low status and to change his status at will. Shortly after this he got a job he wanted, which he has held successfully for over five years at the time of writing.

Exercises such as status games reveal the politics of everyday life and give us a sense of power through understanding them, and a sense of control where before we may have had none.

Status Games
Pecking Order

Four players come out and stand in a line. No 1 is the boss, No 2 is the next in pecking order and so on. No 2 must be respectful to No 1 and call him or her sir or madam and so on down to No 4, who is the underdog. Each player can only speak to the next player. No 1 initiates orders which get sent down the line. No 4 inevitably spends his time finding excuses why nothing can be done.

(A great example of this is the classic sketch from *The Frost Report*, which must be late 60s or early 70s – wow, how years vanish! – with John Cleese as an upper-class gent, Ronnie Barker as middle class and little Ronnie Corbett as the worker.)

1: Get me a cup of tea, Hudson.

2: Tea for sir.

3: Sir wants a cup of tea.

4: A what?

3: Cup of tea, you oaf.

4: Let me get this right. Are you asking me to get you a cup of tea?

1: What's taking so long?

2: I'll just check, sir. No 3, where's the tea?

3: It's No 4, sir, he's so slow.

4: I am not slow. I have never been slow. I am deeply insulted.

3: Move your arse and get a cup of tea.

4: That's done it. I'm not moving till you apologise.

1: Look here, where's my tea?

2: Sorry, sir; sorry. No 3, get the tea or get on your bike.

3: Yes, sir; yes, sir. Get the tea now, No 4.

4: I've got to boil the water first.

3: Well boil it then.

4: The kettle's broken isn't it?

3: Well get a new one then.

4: Can't do that, not without a requisition order in triplicate signed by the boss.

And so on.

VARIATION
Same scenario but Nos 1, 2 and 3 have balloons with which they can hit the next one down on the head. No 4 just has to defend himself with wit!

Master and Servant Games

These games are great fun – this relationship appears in classic comedies going way back in theatre. The Joseph Losey movie *The Servant,* where the very efficient, seemingly low-status servant (Dirk Bogarde, playing against type) gradually takes over from the master (James Fox, according to type), is a classic of the ultimate status transaction. There are innumerable ways of playing with this relationship and here are a few:

Servant on the Hop

In this game the master finds fault with everything the servant says or does. The servant accepts the master's statement and then has the task of talking himself out of the predicament. It's a version of Creative Excuses.

Master: Hudson! Why is there no sugar in my coffee?

Servant: In response to your desire to slim, sir.

Master: Hudson, why are my trousers in this disgusting state?

Servant: Mrs Bridges and I trampled all over them yesterday sir, to assist you in your wish to dress like a hippy for Mr Jack's wedding.

And so on.

Servant in Trouble

In this game the servant always keeps himself in the wrong.

Master: Hudson! Where are my chocolate biscuits?

Servant: I'm afraid I ate them all, sir.

Master: You ate them all?

Servant: Every single lovely one, sir.

Servant Getting Himself into Trouble

Master: What do you mean you ate all my biscuits?

Servant: All three packets, sir.

Master: All three packets?

Servant: And the ice cream, sir.

Or:

Master: Hudson you've done it this time.

Servant: Oh no, sir! Not the bed, sir.

Master: Bed? What about the bed?

Servant: She dragged me onto it and pulled all my clothes off, sir. I couldn't stop her.

Master: How dreadful. I'll sack the woman immediately. Who perpetrated this foul deed?

Servant: Er — your wife, sir.

Trading Places

Master: Hudson, come in, old boy, and sit down; sit in my chair.

Servant: In...er...your chair, sir?

Master: I want your advice, actually.

Servant: My...er...advice, sir?

Master: Make yourself at home, Hudson. Have a drink. What will you have?

Servant: Er…I'm not used to drinking, sir.

Master: Come on, man, make up your mind for God's sake. Relax, will you? You look like a pregnant rabbit.

Servant: Most awfully sorry, sir.

Master: And don't call me 'sir'. Call me 'Dinkie'.

Servant: Er…yes, sir, I mean…er, Dinkie…sir.

And so on.

The fun is in allowing the scene to change and develop, while the relative status of the characters is maintained, even though the roles are nominally reversed. We just know that the servant only has to put a foot wrong and the master will revert to type; and yet, who knows, the servant may just manage to get the better of the exchange in the end.

King and Servants

This is a fierce game and a lot can be learned from it. But be warned, it pushes many people's buttons!

One player is king or queen. He or she sits in front of the group on the throne and 'owns' all the space, the air and everything in the room, even the servants. The other players are servants and their job is to serve the king or queen.

This game is about respect, obedience, honour and right use of space. The servants must serve and honour the king or queen, who must rule justly and fairly, and there are strict rules as to how to do this correctly.

One by one, the servants approach the throne and offer a service. The slightest infraction or imposition and the king 'mock-shoots' them dead. The king may also call for a servant to do something and the servant must obey instantly.

The art, as the servant, is in learning to survive, and therefore learning the ability to play truly low status without even a hint of mocking. The art of being king or queen is in being utterly truthful in one's response to the servant's actions, without letting any personal feelings whatsoever influence you. You must be utterly fair, too, and know why you kill any servant; if you do it just for fun, the facilitator terminates your kingship.

The servant must be available, yet not intrusive, serve yet not be servile. Space is very important and there is a 'correct' space between the servant and the king. Too close and the servant infringes the king's space, too far and the king is inconvenienced. Either way the servant is shot!

In this way participants learn how to use the space. The servant should speak respectfully, yet clearly and without hesitation. A bumbling servant is no good to a king and lets the king's status down. A servant is there to elevate the king's status at all times.

As facilitator you need to monitor the king or queen and demote them if they are not true to the energy of the moment.

Be sure after this game to have time for feedback and sharing.

Slave and Master

In this variation the whole group can be involved at once. As it may press a lot of buttons, make sure to leave time for feedback and sharing.

The group splits into pairs and nominates themselves/each other as either slave or master. The slave then has to do whatever the master dictates until the leader calls for a change over, when the slaves become the masters and vice-versa.

To prevent unreasonable demands from the master, the slave can refuse a command which he 'really can't do' and having said 'I really can't do that!' a slave/master switch takes place.

One of the most interesting things about this game is how difficult people find it to think up things for the slave to do (i.e. how difficult many people find it to play high status).

All theatre improvisations benefit from an awareness of what status you and your partner(s) are playing. In *The Human Zoo* (1969), Desmond Morris gives ten golden rules for people who are number ones. He says they apply to all leaders, from baboons to presidents.

1. You must clearly display the trappings, postures and gestures of dominance.

2. In moments of active rivalry you must threaten your subordinates aggressively.

3. In moments of physical challenge you (or your delegates) must be able to forcibly overpower your subordinates.

4. If a challenge involves brain rather than brawn, you must be able to outwit your subordinates.

5. You must suppress squabbles that break out between your subordinates.

6. You must reward your immediate subordinates by permitting them to enjoy the benefits of their high ranks.

7. You must protect the weaker members of the group from undue persecution.

8. You must make decisions concerning the social activities of your group.

9. You must reassure your extreme subordinates from time to time.

10. You must take the initiative in repelling threats or attacks arising from outside your group.

It is interesting to compare ex-prime ministers/presidents from this perspective. In the UK, the last full king/queen was probably Lady Margaret Thatcher, who understood the stuff of power very well. She was followed by John Major, who was definitely not a 'king' type, and then Tony Blair who was…well that is a question I leave for you. In the USA, Ronald Reagan was kingly and possibly so too was George Bush Senior. Bill Clinton was something else. And then we've had George Bush Junior – more a boy than a king? Or was that his camouflage? Was there a cunning operator under the mask? Then Obama. Who is boss there, I wonder? Well, I'll leave that as an open question.

To raise our consciousness we first have to make these transactions conscious, then we can begin to learn to live and interact without being ruled unconsciously by them. Our 'great work' as humans is to learn to live and relate through unconditional love, and thus to get beyond status issues and domination by our lower self; to get beyond jealousy, envy, avarice, attachments, expectations, judgements, comparisons and the need for approval. To achieve this level of being may be a daunting prospect, but it all begins with awareness of our motives and of the real meanings of our actions.

eight
DANCE GAMES

Dance is a primal activity. All the ancient cultures used ceremonial dance to bond their tribe or village socially and to practise changing their individual states of consciousness to a more collective sense of oneness. By taking play into dance and using evocative music to help the mood of the moment, a group can shift levels of openness and cohesion very easily.

Mirror Dance

Many people know this one!

Everyone has a partner; one partner is the dancer and the other partner is the mirror.

This sounds very simple, but there are catches.

So many of us are trained to be so judgemental and critical, self-doubting and self-negating, stuck firmly in left-brain thinking, that if you set this up too rigidly you will find people trying to mirror exactly and getting anxious as to whether they are 'doing it right'! The very poison we are trying to lead people away from returns, and we are enslaved yet again. It is essential to stress that a structure is only a structure and that it is the essence of the mirror that we are after, not the duplicate. Done in the right way, it is a gentle, freeing exercise in relating through movement. Done in the wrong way, it is a source of anxiety.

I remember the first time I participated in this dance exercise in the 70s, the leader was standing outside the group like a judge/critic/father/mother figure, inducing a feeling of being watched which led to an inner dialogue of self-doubt. It was not a very freeing experience. (And a wonderful example of projection on my part!)

This is one thing as a provocative exercise for a process group where the leader may want to make it push participants' buttons, but it is quite the opposite in a Play-World group, where I want everyone to have an experience of getting beyond their enslavement by a doubting self-consciousness. I make a point of joining in, with or without a partner, so I am not on the outside and do not become the participants' 'father'. (I get enough of people's projections without setting myself up for it!)

Then partners swop roles after one or two minutes and then perhaps swop back once more each way. Then I ask all the couples to allow themselves to dance interactively without either of them leading.

I find it good to vary the music, avoiding anything with a familiar beat like rock or disco. Light classical, New Age meditation music, Malaysian or Peruvian are excellent, also Scott Joplin rags, Indian sitar music; anything that does not provoke an habitual response, but calls for greater creativity.

Counterpoint Dance

This is a variation on the Mirror Dance, but the partner's aim is to dance as a counterpoint to the leader. The movements of the dancer will elicit a response, a counterpoint reaction.

Snakes (or Trains)

Ask everyone to team up with three, four or five others and come into line, one behind the other. The person in front is the leader and begins with a movement. The others mirror the movement and follow like a snake. After a minute or two, blow a whistle/ bang a gong and the leader goes to the back of the snake and the second in line becomes the new leader.

Touch Dance

Invite everyone to touch their partner somewhere – back to back, toe to toe, little finger to little finger.

The dance then simply involves staying in contact and letting the contact move through many parts of the body.

This is good for us British, who are in the habit of not touching.

VARIATION

Ask each couple to find another couple and each one to keep in touch with the other three people while continuing the dance. Then join up with another four, making a group of eight. With luck, chaos and laughter will reign from then on.

Elephant Rub

In pairs, everyone stands back to back, and rubs their backs against each other, imagining they are elephants rolling in the mud.

Put on the weirdest music you can find and let it roll for about 30 seconds to a minute.

Gentle Dances to Make Heartful Contact

Hands Dance

Ask everyone to close their eyes, turn around once or twice, put their hands out in front of them and gently walk forward until they find another pair of hands. Then feel the hands; let them be playful, joyful hands. After a minute or two, keeping eyes closed, bid farewell to these hands and find another pair. Now let your hands be caring, loving hands. The leader partners up those who don't find another pair of hands.

Shoulders

Bid farewell to these hands and, again, keeping your eyes closed, find yet another pair of hands. Now let your hands find your partner's shoulders. Gently massage each other's shoulders.

Face

This game is only if the group is sufficiently open and relaxed.

Gently let your hands move up from your partner's shoulders to their face.

Gently and caringly feel their face.

Let your face be felt.

This is a delightful progression to guide a group to a feeling of intimacy in a non-threatening way. Having the eyes closed helps, and if accompanied by low light or preferably candlelight, it is even better. Soft and mellow New Age music without much of a specific rhythm helps too (see Resources for music suggestions).

Finger-Tips Dance

Partners touch a finger-tip to a finger-tip.

Let a dance happen.

Elbows Dance

Focus on the elbows. Let a dance happen, and elbow dance with another person's elbow.

This one works well with disco music or music with a beat of some kind.

Energy Exchange Dance

Partners dance with each other as if exchanging energy, not touching, but letting each partner's energy affect the other.

Use disco music or anything with a strong beat.

A dance is an energy exchange, anyway. One of the purposes of this game is to overcome the reluctance of men to dance with other men. Women dancing with women is no problem, but the conditioning against men dancing with men is so much stronger. If the group is unbalanced male to female (which is often the case), and I want to get everyone dancing, I call it an energy exchange, not just a dance – even though it amounts to the same thing!

Animal Dance

Close your eyes. Think of your favourite childhood animal. Become that animal. Open your eyes and let the animal 'dance you'.

Find another 'animal' to be your partner.

Enjoy an animal dance!

Feet Dance

Look at your feet and let your feet move.

What is the feeling in your feet? What do they want to express? Let your feet dance until they find another pair of feet to partner.

This can be just a very simple foot dance, or it can become a spectacular, crazy happening! Get everyone to really concentrate on their feet, to look at their feet (and not at the rest of their partner), and then get them into groups of three, five, or even seven, according to the overall size of the group.

Put on good 'foot music', like Ravel's 'Bolero', and tell them that they are becoming monsters and their feet are uncontrollable and are taking them on a journey.

It all depends on the mood of the moment, but I have experienced amazing energy release and creative chaos happening with this simple structure. Low light or candlelight helps encourage people to let go.

Dances to Empower People to Lead
The Dolphin Dance (from Gabrielle Roth)
This is a very simple dance but has great potential.

Bring everyone to one end of the room and tell them that you are going to teach them to dance like dolphins (or that you would do that, except you can't because dolphins have superior faculties to humans!). Dolphins can dance together in perfect harmony due to their sonic radar, but we mere humans need to have someone to follow in order to achieve a dancing unity.

The structure is that someone comes out to the front and spontaneously creates a simple and repetitive dance step which they dance to the other end of the room. It works much better if it doesn't change and is in rhythm with the music. The group mirrors the dance and follows in the leader's footsteps. Then at the other end of the room, someone else steps out as leader and leads everyone back to the first end, and so on.

A good leadership test is to look around when you get to the end and see what you have created as the other dancers come towards you. If your movement was clear and simple to follow, you will have created harmony. If not, you will probably have produced chaos.

One of the great things about this dance is that everyone who wants to, gets a chance to be leader. When leading, it is a good idea to come out to the front of the group without a preconceived idea of what you are going to do. Spend a moment feeling the rhythm and let a movement come 'through' you spontaneously. Let it settle into a steady repetitive action, and then lead off down the room.

This is also an exercise in letting your body dance and not trying to create something clever and impressive. 'Clever' dances don't work, which is useful feedback. The more one can lose oneself within the movement, the better the dance will be. It is about focus and intent and being in the moment.

This is a very powerful dance and can develop an extraordinary feeling of group cohesion, a very tribal feeling. It will also show you those who stay stuck in ego patterns.

Dance Leadership Around the Circle

A simple structure starting in a circle. The leader begins a simple dance step to the music. Like the Dolphin Dance, it needs to be repetitive and easy to follow. The group follows. After half a minute or so the leadership is passed to the next person, who changes the dance to her own step, and the group follows the new leader. The leadership moves around so that everyone gets to be leader in turn.

This is a nice, simple little warm up, which combines exercise with an experience of leadership and avoids the tendency to the mechanistic movements of aerobics.

Changing Dance

Form a standing circle. Have some good rhythmic music playing.

One person goes into the centre and dances her dance. When she has expressed herself, she takes the dance to another member of the circle, who copies it and takes it into the centre while the first person replaces them in the circle. The new person explores the dance she has inherited and gradually, organically, lets it become her own and then takes it to another member of the circle, and so on. This is really a musical version of Changing Movements (see Chapter 4).

Group Theatre Exercises
Disco Dancers

You need a tape of music of all one beat. It can be disco numbers or rock 'n' roll, 20s jazz, African drum music, reggae or anything with a good rhythm. I have used Ravel's 'Bolero' and a delightful New Age music piece called 'The Fairy Ring' by Mike Rowland.

After putting the music on, ask everyone to dance alone and find a movement that the music draws out of them at that moment.

When everyone has found a movement, ask them to join with a partner and teach their movement to the partner. Then they partner up again, in fours now, and teach both movements to their new partners.

(There are then groups of four, each with a basis of four movements.)

Now give them about 10–15 minutes to create a dance piece lasting about two to four minutes, using the movements. Finally, ask them to perform the results for the whole group.

I like to make the rules flexible.

'Leo, do we have to use these movements, or can we alter them?'

'Yes!'

'Leo, do we have to have four movements, or can we have less or more?'

'Definitely yes!'

Sometimes I tell them most seriously and authoritatively, 'You *must* do it exactly the way I have told you, unless you choose to do it in any other way'. It often takes a moment for the penny to drop!

This structure gives everyone the opportunity and encouragement to co-create something together in which everyone makes a contribution. At 'beginners level' it is good to give them about 7 to 15 minutes, but it can be valuable to give much more time to a well warmed-up and inventive group. You will sense when they're ready, and the process has gone as far as it will go naturally.

A good way to help people around the issues of anxiety – performance anxiety is a big thing for many – is to change your mind when they are ready to perform and say you're not going to see the dances, and then to introduce the Dolphin Dance or some other structure instead, or just put on some completely different music for free dancing. Then, when they are distracted from what they have been practising – and getting anxious about – and are relaxed, (and have finished hitting you over the head!), you spring it on them!

When appropriate, it can be very useful to follow this with group-sharing about the experience.

West Side Story – Clans' Dance
(thanks to Denise Taylor)

Get everybody walking around endeavouring to look really cool! A good way to emphasise this is to get them to walk around in a really uncool and depressed way, and then switch to 'walking cool', with a touch of pride in themselves, lengthening the steps a little.

Walking around, find your 'street' movement, a movement that defines your personal power, and then seek the others of your clan and walk around together. The leader encourages the group into sub-groups of about five to eight people, and then gets one group at a time to walk across the diagonal of the room from one corner to the other. Then, repeat lengthening the steps a bit more into a jazz walk. Next, they walk out to eight beats, then jump around/freak out/whoop-it-up for eight beats and then move on to the opposite corner on the last eight beats. On their last beat another clan starts across from another corner, and so on.

Start slowly and speed up until they can do it in the rhythm you want, and then add music. Some good rock music like Michael Jackson or Madonna is good for this, with a beat that suits stepping out.

Finally, get the whole thing in sync. Say you have four groups: Group A (i.e. the group that is in corner A) crosses diagonally to corner C, group B crosses to corner D while group C moves quietly to corner A ready to begin their turn the moment group B completes. Likewise, group D moves to corner B ready to follow group C.

Thus all groups start from corners A and B. This solves the problem of them getting in each other's way. If you didn't quite follow this, don't worry – it works in practice!

Once they have all got the idea, turn the music up and really encourage them to put all they've got into it!

Tribal Gathering

Create a tribal feeling, perhaps with some chanting, call and response chanting, Dolphin Dancing and dancing to drums. Use live music if you have anyone to play, recorded if not. Gabrielle Roth makes wonderful tapes of drum music (see Resources).

Divide the participants into sub-groups of about five to eight people.

The task is to create their tribe with its name, chant, dance, totem (which can be as simple as a drawing), creation myth/ poem, and to find their chief, shaman, elder, storyteller, singers and warriors.

Tell them to create a piece of theatre which tells the story of their own dreamtime – the myth of their creation – including how they were given their name, and how their chant, dance and totems came to them. When they are ready, and this one may take quite a long time in preparation, they imagine they are at a pow-wow; each tribe introduces themselves to the others, performs their dance, tells their myth, shows their totem and so on.

For this it is good to supply face paints, paper and crayons, Blu-tack, bits of material, bits of wood, some feathers, odds and ends and all sorts of oddments. It's amazing how creative people can be when given this sort of opportunity.

A 1980s participant, Bill Downey, gave the following feedback:

This is a wonderful happening and it shows very clearly how, given human/tribal sized-groups, creativity naturally flourishes. Many people readily fall into tribal roles – add to the ones above dancers, drummers, poets, gardeners, artefact makers – and begin to see the areas in which their natural talents lie. In a tribal society such talents would be spotted and encouraged by kindly elders. Not so in our society, where we can easily get programmed to think that unless we play the violin as well as Menuhin, we are useless and without talent It is deeply tragic how many people come to feel they lack any creative talent. In truth it is just lying underneath the surface, unexpressed in our alienating society. Tribal night shows very clearly the deep longing people have for a real community and the potential for creative happiness and expression that lies dormant in them.

Musical Groups

Ask for suggestions of types of musical groups/bands, e.g. rock group/country and western/punk /reggae/rap/Gregorian chanters/a cappella singers/opera singers/soul/jazz/choir boys and girls/ heavy metal and so on.

Divide the group into sub-groups of four to eight people. Bring each sub-group forward and ask the others to suggest a musical style for them and a first line of a song.

Give them 10 to 20 minutes to prepare and then invite them to perform their song for everyone else.

This can produce the most wonderful hilarious nonsense and is a structure which elicits great creativity.

nine

THE BLAMER, THE PLACATER, THE COMPUTER AND THE DISTRACTER

I first met the late Virginia Satir at the One Earth Gathering at Findhorn in 1977. Much later, when I was working on my MA at Antioch University in San Francisco, she came there to give a workshop on family therapy, her speciality. She was a delightful lady, a very warm person and a very skilled therapist. The workshop was composed of about 50 people, and though she only worked directly with a few, it felt as though she had done healing on all of us.

In this chapter I have used the categories which she used there: the Blamer, the Placater, the Computer and the Distracter. She coined them, and I use them extensively to illustrate typical ways of responding neurotically to life. Some of the most amusing and most healing creative theatre we have done has been based on these archetypes. See if you recognise aspects of yourself!

The Satir Categories

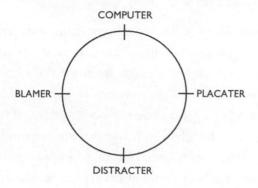

The Placater (or 'Do-Gooder' or 'Pleaser')

Inner dialogue: 'I agree with everything... Whatever you want is okay, I am just here to make you happy.'

Body: Placating and pleading pose.

Movement: Wringing hands.

Inside feelings: 'I am helpless and hopeless, without you I am nothing.'

Note: This role reminds me of that ghastly song performed by Engelbert Humperdinck/Elvis and others:

There goes my reason for living (*really?*), there goes the one of my dreams.

There goes my only possession (*yuk*), there goes my everything.

Talk about giving away your power! Truly an archetypal song of worthlessness!

Status: Low or super low!

Archetype: Patrick and Polly Please.

The Placater always talks in an ingratiating way, trying to please, apologising, never disagreeing, no matter what. He's a 'yes man'. He talks as though he could do nothing for himself; he must always get someone to approve of him. A big help in doing a good placating job is to think of yourself as lucky just to be alive, and that you are responsible for everything that goes wrong. Naturally, you will agree with any criticism made of you and perhaps even encourage it. You are, of course, grateful for the fact that anyone even talks to you, no matter what they say or how rude they are. After all, who are you to object?

Be the most syrupy, martyrish, boot-licking person you can be! Think of yourself as being physically down on one knee, wobbling a bit, putting one hand out in a begging fashion, and be sure to have your head up so your neck will hurt and your eyes become strained so that in no time at all you begin to get a headache. When you talk in this position, your voice will be whiny and squeaky; you keep your body in such a lowered position that you don't have enough air to produce a full, rich tone. You will be saying 'yes' to everything, no matter what you feel or think.

The Blamer (or 'Hostile' or 'Fart')

Inner dialogue: 'I disagree and you're wrong. What is the matter with you? You never do anything right.'

Body: Blames and asserts. 'I am the boss around here and I count the most.'

Inside feelings: 'I'm a failure and I'm lonely but I'm damned if I'll let anyone see.'

Movement: Pusher.

Status: High.

Archetype: Bert and Bessie Blamer.

The Blamer is a fault-finder, a dictator, a boss. He acts superior, and seems to be saying, 'If it weren't for you, everything would be all right.' The internal feeling is one of tightness in the muscles and internal organs. Meanwhile, the blood pressure is increasing. The voice is hard, tight and often shrill and loud.

Good blaming requires you to be as loud and tyrannical as you can be. Cut everyone and everything down. A great model is Basil Fawlty, John Cleese's wonderful invention.

As a Blamer, think of yourself pointing a finger accusingly and start your sentences with, 'You never do this/ that right, it's always your fault', or, 'Why do you always/ never...', and so on. Don't bother about an answer – that is quite unimportant. The Blamer is much more interested in throwing his weight around than in finding out about anything.

When you are blaming you will find yourself breathing in tight little spurts, or holding your breath altogether, because your throat muscles are tight. Have you ever seen a really first-rate blamer whose eyes were bulging, neck muscles and nostrils standing out, who was getting red in the face, and whose voice sounded like someone shovelling coal?

Stand with one hand on your hip, extend the other with your index finger pointing straight out. Screw up your face, curl your lips, flare your nostrils, and let rip. Call people names, criticise everything in sight, blame everyone around for everything, be obnoxious. Let the Blamer in you come out. (Then apologise and placate like mad before you lose all your friends!)

The Computer (or Zombie)

Inner dialogue: Rational, logical, thinking, sensible. 'I think, therefore I am.'

Body: Computes. 'I'm cool, calm and collected.'

Inside feelings: 'I feel inadequate and vulnerable but I must hide it at all costs.'

Movement: Rubbing (tends to rub hands on his clothes, chair arms and so on).

Status: Most Computers play high status, but occasionally you may stumble across one with a creepy, low status.

Archetype: Peter Plan and Penelope Plan.

The Computer is very correct, very reasonable, with no semblance of feeling showing, if at all possible. He is Mr Cool, Calm and Collected. He could be compared to an actual computer or dictionary. The body feels dry, often cool and dissociated. The voice is a dry monotone and the words are usually abstract.

When you act as a computer, use the longest words possible, however unnecessary, even if you are not sure of their meanings. You will at least kid yourself that you sound intelligent. After a bit, no one will be listening anyway. To prepare for this role, imagine that your spine is a long, heavy steel rod reaching from the nape of your neck to your buttocks, and you have a ten-inch-wide collar around your neck. Keep everything about you as motionless as possible, including your mouth. Let your hands and arms feel like lead, slow to move.

When you are a Computer, your voice will naturally go dead because you have no feelings about anything. Your mind is intent on being right about everything, choosing the right word, never making a mistake, being invulnerable.

The really sad thing about this role is that it represents a goal for some people; say the right words, show no feeling, don't react, keep your real self hidden, let the world see only the mask.

The Distracter (or Space Cadet)

Inner dialogue: 'I'm really irrelevant but I've got to survive somehow.' (The words make little sense and hop from one subject to another without much sense of continuity.)

Body: Angular. Going in several directions at once.

Inside feelings: 'I'm unloved. Nobody cares for me. I don't belong anywhere.'

Movement: Flicker. Tends to keep flicking imaginary or real dust from clothes, anything from anywhere.

Status: Low, but sometimes covered up with an attempt to play high.

Archetype: Cindy and Steve Space.

Whatever the Distracter says or does is irrelevant to what anyone else is saying or doing. He never makes a response to the point. His internal feeling is one of dizziness; life is pretty confusing most of the time. The voice is usually out of tune with the words and can often be singsong and go up or down without reason.

When you play this role, think of yourself as a lopsided top, constantly spinning, but never quite stable, never knowing where you are going and not really knowing when you get there – if indeed you do – because you are too busy moving your mouth, body, arms and legs to notice. Make sure you are never quite to the point with your words. Ignore other people's questions or, better still, come back with one of your own on a different subject. Take a piece of imaginary fluff off someone's clothes, or untie or tie up shoelaces at the wrong moment.

Think of your body as going off in several directions at once. Put your knees together in an exaggerated knock-kneed fashion. This will bring your buttocks out and make it easy for you to hunch your shoulders and have your arms and hands going in opposite directions.

At first this role may seem quite easy and fun, but after a few minutes of constant non-connection you may get an acute feeling of loneliness and purposelessness.

Fun with the Satir Categories

Warm Up

As a warm up for this, I often divide the group into four so that one sub-group can act out each category. I then get in the middle and become a Blamer. I try to look as if I'm having a 'turn' so some people will think it is almost real, not just an act. I become progressively more unpleasant and take on the physical attitudes, vocal qualities and pushy movements of the Blamer character and start blaming everyone in sight for whatever I can think of at that moment.

I imagine myself tight in the throat, desperate in the gut, with bulging neck and red nose. I pretend to be Basil Fawlty. I accuse, make disparaging remarks, insult people's dress, kid people (especially anyone I know well) until I get a reaction. Usually this comes very quickly, and then wonderful, spontaneous theatre happens.

I soon see which group has the most blaming energy at that moment and designate them the Blamers.

I then make them fully responsible for my terrible, gross behaviour as I switch to Placater and apologise profusely for all the frightful things I have just said. I simply cannot understand what came over me and how I could have said such things, and I am abjectly sorry. I usually get on my knees at this point, telling everyone I really hope they are enjoying the workshop (playshop), and I do hope it is okay and I am so glad they haven't walked out yet, but there is still time if they would like to, because after all it's really so kind of them to come and support me, and what would I do if they weren't there? Well, I'd just be alone and I'd probably cry, but don't worry about me because I'm not worth it. I'll do anything to please – just tell me what to do… I know I have nothing to teach and don't know anything worth knowing anyway. I'll do anything you want, just tell me what you would like…

Even though this is role-play, it brings some very interesting reactions. The authority figure is suddenly without authority. The 'king' has no 'clothes'. Some people suffer from quite a degree of insecurity if I do this. Workshop leaders tend to get a quite undeserved degree of high, at times even guru, status, and this is a great way to break that mirage. It is painful to fall from a high pedestal so better to make it small!

I finally come back to myself and designate the most placatory group as the Placaters. Then without any warning I become serious and intellectual. I pretend to be an accountant/internet nerd and become highly rational and devoid of feelings, a true Computer. I use long words and adopt the stance of the Computer. If anyone responds with even a hint of feeling, I insist that they immediately stop that nonsense and think and consider matters sensibly like 'proper' (British!) people. I speak in long words and look into the distance as I'm talking. Soon people start talking back to me in a similar fashion and we interface and compete for long-windedness. Sometimes an almost sensible nonsense discussion ensues. The appropriate group becomes the Computers.

I then get distracted about time, forget what we are doing, talk about the weather or the state of the nation or my desire for a cup of tea. I take up the physical stance of the Distracter. All sorts of spontaneous distracting things happen, as by then everyone in the room is conversant with the game. The last group becomes the Distracters.

Development

The next step is for each group to take up the appropriate stance and behaviour and then to walk around feeling that they are inside their character/the character is inside them, adopting the body movement, saying the words most personally appropriate and really getting into the feeling of that part of themselves.

Then I ask them to mingle and meet others of all categories, and interact and see what happens. A lot of energy gets released at this point, and we have a lot of fun. I then invite everyone to choose the category they now feel most at home with, and re-form the groups in that way. Again, in their self-chosen role, I ask them to mingle and interact and see what it feels like.

Theatre Pieces

Step three is to create theatre pieces. The ideal group size is about four to seven people, so if one group is too large, form it into two groups doing that particular category separately, or if it's too small, just do the three categories which have evoked the most response. Arrange the sub-groups and then ask them to sit down and share in turn their individual feelings of the category they have elected to play. For example: What does it mean to be a Placater? When do you placate in your life? How often do you give your power away and get trodden on, when you would have done better to stand up for yourself? What does it cost you personally to live your life as a pleaser-person? Are you buying 'being liked' at expense to yourself?

When they have shared about their issues, ask them to think how they can dramatise this in a short piece of up to five minutes which encapsulates the essence of the main issue that has surfaced. It is good not to give too much time to rehearsing, as all that is needed is a framework within which the words can be improvised at the time. It creates more spontaneity to go into it in a state of moderate unreadiness. The Blamers won't like it of course, the Placaters will see it as their fault anyway, the Computers will point out that they could have been better had they only been given more time and the Distracters won't notice. The nearer the piece is to real experience, the better. One true piece speaks volumes to a room full of people.

Case Study

Many years ago at a Play-World Saturday evening event, we were playing these categories and my colleague Trisha Wood was in the Placaters group. She felt that this was a big issue for her and that she had lost a lot in her life through being overly nice and super accommodating. On this night the sketch that came out was nauseatingly wonderful. Trisha played one of two daughters who both had the same boyfriend. She very insistently gave away her boyfriend to her sister: 'No dear, you take him. He's much too good for me. You'll be better for him. I'm not good enough for anyone. I only want his happiness and yours. I'll make the wedding cake and wash up at the reception.' The sketch went on like that until – and this had not been planned beforehand – the placating became more and more competitive and intense, the volume rose and suddenly it all erupted into glorious rage – and the truth!

Trish said later that she felt so sick at seeing that part of herself so clearly that she stopped placating – not exactly overnight, but when she found herself doing it, automatically that scenario flashed before her eyes and she was able to override her behaviour. She gradually modified that pattern and her life noticeably changed for the better.

Victim, Persecutor, Rescuer and Therapist (Another Variation on the Same Theme)

The Victim

The moment we blame others or complain, we are playing victim. To avoid playing victim means we must take responsibility for ourselves and our life. That's a tall order. Most of us have been brought up to blame and complain. Many people play victim a lot of the time and, perhaps, rather more than they would wish to admit. The great value in this role-play is to bring to consciousness this tendency. Note: The Victim is the most powerful position of these three. The Victim manipulates and controls and arranges his own martyrdom. A persecutor needs someone to persecute, a rescuer needs someone to rescue, a therapist someone to 'therap', but a victim can manage all on his own!

When playing victim, first of all think of all the circumstances which you could possibly interpret as being against you. Trains and buses which make you late, restaurants which overcharge, service which is slack. And then there are the people who have victimised you – parents who have made you what you are, bosses who made you work far too hard and paid you far too little, lovers who've taken what they wanted and then discarded you like an empty beer can, children who want you to die so they can inherit your money, people who have pinched your best ideas and called them their own...the list is endless. Get to feel really bad about yourself and fiendishly angry about all the frightful things *other people* are responsible for in your life. Think of the people who have persecuted you and made you out to be wrong when you knew you were right. Revel in the sheer awfulness of it all. Say out loud the phrase which encapsulates your terrible underdog life: 'Poor me, they really see me coming', 'I only have to pop my head above water to have it chewed off!' Find the phrase which is most meaningful to you and say it as a Tragedy Queen or King. Go right over the top and let the world know just how badly you have been treated. Perhaps you feel that even God is against you, that the Universe is just waiting to chop you down to size. Well, now is your chance to complain about it, to let the world know!

Everybody walk around, mingle and find the posture and walk that exemplifies the Victim. Feel inside yourself for the core of this awful feeling. Check out your voice and the position of your neck. How long could you spend boring someone to death telling them how many myriad awful things have been done to you? What would be your catch-phrase? Find someone and really let them know just how badly life has treated you. List the awful hand life has dealt you, and don't spare them the grimy details. Make quite sure they really know it is *you* and no one else who has suffered these appalling indignities, and don't forget just how much worse yours are than theirs. If they keep on trying to butt in with their minor little quibbles about pathetic little setbacks, don't listen to their rubbish, just keep on telling them about your definitive suffering until they realise it is *you* that has truly suffered.

The Persecutor

Every victim needs a persecutor. Indeed, every victim creates a persecutor, and vice-versa. Now it is time to find the Persecutor inside you. Look at all these snivelling little Victims, don't they deserve what they get?

Wretched little people creeping about the world, moaning, complaining, whining, fault-finding, boring you to death with their petty little concerns. Wouldn't you just like to tell them how pathetic and feeble they are? After all, how can any sensible person with any self-respect go through life like that? How can anyone with even a grain of intelligence be so utterly irresponsible about themselves? Ridiculous, cringing little wets!

Find your posture and your walk as a Persecutor, the position of your hands and the sound of your voice. If this role is unfamiliar, feel the rage inside. Feel the powerlessness too – yes, persecutors feel powerless just like victims, but they handle the feeling by aggressing instead of whining – so let yourself feel this helplessness, and remember that if you are going to get anywhere in the world, it will be by climbing over someone else's back. In this role it is good to be bad. You can say those cutting remarks that you may have never dared say in real life. You can drop put-downs like Father Christmas drops presents. You can creatively insult anyone if it will give you a moment's satisfaction. As a Persecutor you need to make your mark so everyone will know you are not a person to be messed with. If there is anything going here, you are going to get your share first.

Find your catch-phrase: 'I didn't get where I am today being the sort of person who…', 'The world is full of pathetic non-entities', 'It takes a real man like me', 'When I was a boy, we never had…like all the softies of today!' Find the phrase that works for you, which encapsulates the Persecutor in you, perhaps a phrase you have often wanted to say. Well, now is the time to let loose and persecute! Have a ball! Be an insulting pig, let everyone around know you are bigger than they are. If they just happen to start cutting you down, well just give them double what they give you. Don't let any snivelling little creep get the better of you. You are going to win, or else!

The Rescuer

Sometimes we feel that we know best and can help others. We feel that we can do a good deed and rescue others from their own follies. After all, poor unfortunate Victims need someone to rescue them, don't they? And Persecutors need to be helped to see that they don't need to behave badly. Yes, it's time to find the noble, self-sacrificing Rescuer within.

Ask yourself how much good you can do by helping these poor unfortunate people to see the error of their ways, and what loving assistance you can give to the poor unfortunate Victims who seem, over and over again, to bring such suffering down upon their own heads. After all, you know better, don't you?

You can help and advise, and the wise counsel that falls so easily from your lips will surely prevail. People will see reason when they see what a fountain of good sense *you* are. And those Persecutors? They need to be told a thing or two, don't they? They think they are it, but you know it's all just bravado, just showing off. And, furthermore, it's very mean to pick on those more helpless than oneself. They should pick on people their own size if they have to, not on poor unfortunates who already feel victimised.

Find the posture of the Rescuer. Remember that you are there to save these poor people, whether they like it or not. *You* are the Robin Hood of emotional neuroses and *you* are going to bring them the riches of true self-understanding.

Go to it! Do them good; save them; rescue them from their short-sighted stupidity and ignorance. And remember, if they don't like what you are doing, *you know best* and *you* can save them. After all, it's your vocation, and you know how good you are because you can count up how many you have saved already as, naturally, you keep a record.

So, let's hear some heroic martial music as you come triumphantly to the rescue like a knight on a white horse, declaring your catch-phrase: 'I'm here to rescue you from yourself', 'Just let *me*...', 'Take advice from one who knows', 'Let *me* save you'.

Although those are three interlocking archetypal roles, it is possible to add a fourth – Therapist. This is not necessary, as the three roles are complete, in the sense that each one necessitates the other and provides the raw material for it. However, the addition of the role of Therapist can provide a lot of fun, particularly if members of the group are familiar with therapy.

The Therapist

The Therapist is quite unlike the Rescuer, because whereas the latter is determined to do 'good' whether it helps or not, and is doing it for personal prestige and ego boosting, the Therapist is there to reflect the games to the other players. So when a Victim is complaining, the Therapist might observe: 'I notice you feel victimised', or 'I am wondering what you get out of arranging your life to be persecuted so much'. Or, to a Persecutor: 'I wonder what you get out of bullying this person'. And to a Rescuer: 'I am wondering what's in it for you to spend so much effort trying to save this person, particularly when they clearly do not wish to be saved', and so on. These are aggravating statements to be on the receiving end of.

To be a Therapist means that you do not buy into other people's emotional trips; you remain emotionally aloof. You can play this to the hilt, like the other roles, and produce the most wonderfully annoying questions and observations. Your task is to make the other people's games unplayable by showing them up at every opportunity. This role can be played for laughs or for real. There are probably more options with this than the other roles. See if you can find the Therapist within you, how it feels. Build up your character as with the other roles, but remember that unlike the other roles you are to stay centred all the time – if you can!

Ways of Playing

You can do all the same things with these characters as with the Placater, Blamer, Computer and Distracter. Alternatively, here is a different scenario.

Get everybody to walk around and find one of the characters within themselves. Posture first, then walk, voice, phrase, expression.

Then they interact with one or two others. Do this for each role.

Then divide into four sub-groups, one group playing each role.

Mingle and interact for a couple of minutes.

Ask the participants to identify which role they feel most at home with (or you may prefer to ask them which role they would like to work on, to experience). Next, ask them to divide into four sub-groups again, one group for each role, the role being their own choice. They then mingle again and interact. Then ask them what has surfaced for them in the role-play and discuss the issues.

Ask each group to come up with an archetype of their role and for one member to act it out (one or two minutes).

Alternatively, they become a panel and members of the other groups ask them questions which they answer in role.

Or, each group creates a theatre piece to show the meaning of the role and to expose the feelings behind the stereotype being portrayed.

Or, ask one member from each category to come together to form a group. They then create a sketch with each category represented.

What may well happen in the playing is that the roles change. The Knight Rescuer may become a Victim, the Victim may easily start to Persecute, the Persecutor becomes Therapist and the Therapist may become a Rescuer on a white charger! And so on. This is the best kind of outcome as it happens in life.

Emotional Triangle Game

This is an adaptation of a game I learned from the Actors Institute, which sadly seems to be defunct. In the original version the three parts are Love, Anger, Pleading. This game is suitable for a well warmed-up and fairly extrovert group. Don't use it the first night of a beginners' group. It needs players with a measure of confidence, but it can take group energy right up if it is played at the psychologically right moment. It needs to be played at full volume with no holds barred vocally, and no physical violence under any circumstances whatever!

Three participants come out front.

The one in the middle expresses love – unconditional love – no matter what happens or what is said.

The one on the left side expresses anger and has the opportunity to let rip with everything – no holds barred on language. (This game is not suitable for church bazaars!)

The third player is on the other side and expresses pleading. This is a life or death situation, so it's not a matter of 'Please, will you help me?' but 'Heellpppp!'

The scene is like this:

Anger	Love	Pleading

Either: the same three can switch roles till they have experienced all three.

Or: the Pleader goes off, Love moves to Pleading and Anger to Love, and another person from the group comes on stage taking the Anger place. They move across doing each role in turn with a new person joining each round, i.e. first Anger, then Love, then Pleading. (Or you can set it up the other way with Pleading first.)

The three participants go full-tilt all at once. It helps to get the rest of the group to give vocal encouragement! (Those who played only one or two roles at the beginning will circle round to come back on at the end to complete their turn.)

Time: half to one minute, not more.

Prop: Loud whistle or gong to signal beginning and end of each short interaction.

Alternative categories for this game are:

Persecutor	Victim	Rescuer

And:

Blamer	Computer/Distracter	Placater

ten
CLOSING A SESSION

Closing is as important as starting. In many ways, a play session as described in this book is like a dream where the rules of everyday society are changed, where judgements and comparisons are suspended and where extraordinary magical things occur. When the games, dance improvs and drama games are over, people will be ready to relax and dance. If so, turn down the lights, light some candles and put on some appropriate music (no structure).

I remember using the Sister Sledge hit 'We Are Family' many years ago when it was popular. By the end of the evening we felt like a family.

Soundbath

A good structure to follow is a Soundbath.

Call the group together in a standing circle and invite about a fifth to a quarter of the people to go into the centre. They face outwards, link up and close their eyes. Ask the outer circle to join you in bathing them in sound. Start with a single note and then improvise around it. The group members will pick this up and join you in creating a weave of sound. Let it go on for two or three minutes, and when it feels like enough, gently indicate you are bringing it to a close. Invite the people in the centre to exchange with others and repeat.

The final act to honour the dreamspace, as you come to the end of a session, is to bring everyone into the circle (sitting is good for this), turn down the lights, put a candle in the centre and sing together or just be together. Apart from chanting, a very nice thing to do at this point is to hum together.

Hum Circle

As for the Soundbath, invite everyone to join in humming a tone and when the tone is established, to ad-lib harmonies around the base note.

At the end of the evening (or the time spent together) it is necessary to help people to come back to everyday reality, the state of consciousness in which it is safe to drive a car, catch a bus and so on. This is the time to make any announcements, talk about future events and so on. If necessary, do the Chakra Closing exercise below.

Chakra Closing

Sometimes it is necessary to close ourselves down. Here is a simple exercise.

Stretch your arms up above your head and, holding the idea that you are closing yourself down, bring your hands down towards your crown, then down the front of your body, closing your third eye, throat, heart, solar plexus, belly and base. Raise your arms a second time and repeat, covering any other areas that may need closing. Then cross your hands in front of you, making the sign of shutting down over your solar plexus and belly area.

A good mantra before driving is to walk round the car four times, stamping the ground and saying 'I am here now!'

Programming a Play-World Evening Session: a Few Suggestions

These are just a few ways of putting together an evening. It's good to come with an idea of a programme but it's even better to be willing to be spontaneous and change your order of events according to the mood and feeling of the moment. There is no way of knowing beforehand whether you will be faced with a vibrant, willing and raring-to-go group, or a tired and resistant one which will take all your skills to get relaxed and into the energy. Each situation calls for a different programme, and part of a leader's skill is to suss out quickly which games will work best in each set of circumstances.

There are natural waves of energy in groups, which it is vital to keep track of. Often a group will begin with quite high energy, some of which is displaced nervousness, but will follow your lead readily for three-quarters to one hour in active high energy games. At some time it will be just right to tone it down with something like gentle dancing or a trust game. If you do this in the first session, you will be able to raise energy again after a break and it will be better quality energy in the sense that people will be much more relaxed with each other.

Some games I find to be good stand-bys when I want to raise the energy are:

Movement Crescendo and Yes/No followed by Mimicry, Pass the Face and Hot Coals, Machines and Paranoid.

And some dances for engaging low energy or bringing a high-energy group down to a more introspective place are:

Mirror Dance, Counterpoint, Touch, Hands, Shoulders, Finger-Tips.

Or Car Wash, Blind Lead.

Dances to raise group energy are:

Snakes, Elbows, Animal Dance, Energy Exchange and Dolphin Dance.

(If you cannot get a group going with games, go right on to dance and come back to games later.)

Programme Suggestions for an Evening Session

Programme No 1

Circle:

Opening circle

Italian Breathing

Whisper Name Game

Movement Crescendo

Face Pass

Two lines:

Yes/No

Mimicry

Dance:

Mirror Dance

Counterpoint Dance

Snakes

Hands Dance or Shoulder Dance

Dolphin Dance

Free dancing to rhythmic music

Break for refreshments

Dancing to 1920s music

(Hats, scarves and bits and pieces like that are excellent here as props.)

Circle:

Changing Movements

The Meaning of Life

You're Lucky

Theatre:

Paranoid

The Statuary

Interruptions

Freeze

Circle:

Closing circle

Programme No 2
Circle:

Opening circle

Spiral

Name Cushion (short version and then...)

Terrific Teresa

Sound and Movement Round

Pass the Clap

Devils into Angels

Mingling:

Wrong Names

Opposite Emotions

Tag-Freeze

Pat Bottoms

Stop – Go

Circles of five to eight:

Trust Circle (or Car Wash)

Dance:

Mirror Dance

Elephant Rub

Hands Dance

Shoulders Dance

Face Dance

Dance leadership around the circle

Exchange Energy Dance

Break for refreshments

Free dancing

Circle:

    Machines

    Orchestra and Conductor

    Merry-Go-Round

Mingling:

    Never Mind That, Tell Me About...

    Points on the Floor

Groups of four to eight:

    Musical Groups

Dancing and closing circle

Programme No 3

Circle:

    Opening circle

    Moving Circle

Mingling:

    Cocktail Party

    Suspicious

    Anger Release

    Compassion

    Sadness

    Joy

Circle:

    Name Crescendo

    Imaginary Ball Toss

    Face Pass

    Lap Sit

    Knot

    Shoulder Massage

Dance:

    Mirror Dance

    Touch Dance

    Animal Dance

    Snakes

    Feet Dance

    Energy Exchange Dance

    Break for refreshments

    Free dancing

Two lines:

    Yes/No

    Mimicry

    Culinary Insults

Groups of four to eight:

    The Blamer, the Placater, the Computer and the Distracter

Dancing and closing circle

In Conclusion

Play is a natural part of life – just play for no other reason than playing. All children do this naturally. Our ancient ancestors knew this and encouraged their children to play freely without restriction. Unfortunately, in most modern cultures, children get taught out of play before their natural time and guided into 'serious' pursuits such as the mental learning of 'facts'.

In strengthening the Magical Child in each of us adults through creative play, we gain more confidence to be our true selves instead of the culturally conditioned mask. This can help us enormously in the difficult task of healing the Wounded Child. Approaching the therapeutic process from the opposite end, instead of starting with 'what's my problem?/what's wrong with me?', we can start with 'how can I have fun, be myself, relax, laugh, be creative and enjoy life?' As one goes deeply into play, the old hurts can surface and be healed in an atmosphere of openness and trust, where there is no competitiveness, no put-downs, just acceptance, support and unconditional lovingness. This is the most healing environment there is. This is the Magic of Play.

Resources

Books

Brandes, D. and Phillips, W. (1977) *Gamesters' Handbook*. London: Hutchinson.

Castaneda, C. (1972) *Journey to Ixtlan*. Simon and Schuster: New York.

Cousins, N. (1981) *Anatomy of an Illness*. New York: Bantam.

Cohen, D. (2006) *The Development of Play*. Abingdon: Taylor and Francis.

Jeffers, S. (2012) *Feel The Fear and Do It Anyway*. London: Vermilion.

Johnstone, K. (2012) *Impro – Improvisation and the Theatre*. New York: Theatre Arts Books.

LeFevre, D.N. *Playing For The Fun Of It*. Stockholm, Sweden: published by the author.

Masheder, M. (1989) *Let's Play Together*. London: Green Print.

Masters, R. and Houston, J. (1998) *Mind Games*. Delta, IL: The Theosophical Publishing House.

Roth, G. (1998) *Maps to Ecstasy*. Novata, CA: New World Library.

Spolin, V. (1999) *Improvisation for the Theater*. Evanston, IL: Northwestern University Press.

Swimme, B. (1984) *The Universe is a Green Dragon*. Rochester, Vermont: Bear and Company.

Weinstein, M. and Goodman, J. (1980) *Playfair – Everybody's Guide to Non-Competitive Play*. San Luis Obispo, CA: Impact Publishers Inc.

Books by the Author

Rutherford, L. (1994) *Principles of Shamanism*. London: HarperCollins (republished third edition 2014 by Crescent Moon, Kent).

Rutherford, L. (2001/2006) *Shamanic Path Workbook*. London: Piatkus 2001/Suffolk: Arima 2006.

Rutherford, L. (2008) *The View through the Medicine Wheel*. Winchester: O-Books.

Rutherford, L. (2011) *Spirituality versus Religion*. CreateSpace.

Music

It is good to have the widest selection of music available, especially unfamiliar rhythms which move participants to find new expressions in dance. Here is a selection. I have only put details where they are not readily available in record stores. The main thing is to make your own selection from each of the categories, and any other categories I may have left out.

Chants (some quoted in the book)

Leo Rutherford and friends – *Forty-Four Chants – Words and Music*.

A teaching CD for learning chants 'Ancient and Modern' – comes complete with the book of words.

Leo Rutherford and friends – *Turn the World Around*.

Twenty-eight chants and community songs, complete with the book of words.

Both the previously mentioned works are available from the author at £10 (abroad at £13), including postage and packaging.

Visit www.eagleswing.co.uk/shop/ or email Info@eagleswing.org.uk.

Classical

Pachelbel's 'Canon in D' (wonderfully evocative, gentle piece).

Vivaldi – 'The Four Seasons'.

Ravel – 'Bolero'.

Chopin – 'Piano Nocturne'.

Mussorgsky – 'Pictures at an Exhibition'.

Carl Orff – *Carmina Burana*.

Liszt – 'Hungarian Dances'.

'Missa Luba'.

Lloyd Webber – 'Pie Jesu' and 'Benedictus' from *Requiem*.

New Age

Mike Rowland – 'The Fairy Ring'/'Titania the Fairy Queen'.

Tim Wheater – 'The Enchanter'.

John Richardson – 'Spirit of the Redman'.

Tani Senzan, (Shakuhachi flute) – 'Zen Spirit'.

Anthea Gomez – 'Watercolours'.

John Atkins – 'Sea of Dreams'.

Excellent Contemporary Drums

Gabrielle Roth and the Mirrors – 'Waves', 'Bones', 'Trance', 'Ritual', 'Totem'.

Drums of Passion – Olatunji (No 1 – original version is best).

Kodo Drummers of Japan – any selection.

Jazz/Ragtime

Scott Joplin's *Piano Rags*.

Temperance Seven – any selection.

Pasadena Roof Orchestra – any selection.

A selection by Chris Barber, Acker Bilk, Monty Sunshine or similar band of your choice.

Swing

Any selection by Duke Ellington/Benny Goodman/ Artie Shaw/Tommy Dorsey, etc.

Rock 'n' roll 50s/60s style:
> Bill Haley and the Comets – *Greatest Hits*.
> Elvis Presley – any selection.
> The Beatles – any selection.

John Lennon – 'Imagine'.

Wings – 'Let it Be'.

Reggae

Bob Marley and the Wailers – *Exodus*/*Greatest Hits*, etc.
> Two greatest tracks are 'Three Little Birds' and 'One Love'.

African

Miriam Makeba – *Welela*.

Bundu Boys – any selection.

Real Sounds of Africa – any selection.

Meditation

Stephen Russell – *First Orbit – A Taoist Meditation*.

Gregorian chants sung by Benedictine Nuns.

Gyume Tibetan Monks – Tantric Harmonics.

Spirit Sounds – *Dolphin Dreams*.

Frank Perry – *Deep Peace*/*Star Peace* (Tibetan bowls and gongs).

Peruvian Music

Any selection by Incantations (Excellent British group).

Gheorghe Zamfir – 'The Lonely Shepherd' (and other titles).

Rumillajta – 'Hoja de Coca'.

Flight of the Condor (from BBC TV series).

American Indian Flute Music

Robert Mirabal (PO Box 871, Taos, New Mexico 87571, USA) – 'Sys-to-le'.

R. Carlos Nakai – Earth Spirit.

Chants

Forty-Four Chants – Words And Music (CD and booklet).

Turn The World, Around – 28 Chants and Community Songs (CD and booklet).

Available from: Eagle's Wing College of Contemporary Shamanism – www.eagleswing.co.uk (at £10 including postage and packaging).

Greek

Greece Forever (Greek dance music).

Any selection of typical Greek music which evokes holidays in Greece!

Samba/Rumba/Tango/Salsa – the Music of South America

Courses and Workshops

Eagle's Wing College of Contemporary Shamanism.

Workshops and courses run by the author and friends.

www.eagleswing.co.uk.

List of Games

CPI Antony Rowe
Eastbourne, UK
June 20, 2023